ROMANTIC MASSAGE
a step by step guide for
lovers of all ages

SASHA CRAIG-TAYLOR   VTCT, C&G, ITEC

www.romantic-massage.com

ISBN-10: 1477551123
ISBN-13: 978-1477551127

CONTENTS

	Preface	Pg 1
1	Touching Moments	Pg 2
2	Skin – a remarkable organ	Pg 4
3	Taking care of your skin	Pg 6
4	Anyone for a massage?	Pg 8
5	Getting started	Pg 11
6	Essential oils to affect the emotions	Pg 13
7	Basic massage techniques	Pg 15
8	Whole body massage	Pg 18
9	Mini massages: Indian Head Massage	Pg 30
10	Mini massages: foot massage	Pg 38
11	Mini massages: face massage	Pg 43
12	Romantic mutual massage	Pg 47
13	Massage your relationship	Pg 52
14	Heightening your senses	Pg 53
15	Essential oils to enhance your relationship	Pg 54
	About the author	Pg 55

ACKNOWLEDGMENTS

I could never have illustrated this book without the help of my husband and best friend, Mike. He is a professional photographer and his excellent photography brings the text to life. And we would like to thank our photographic models, Eva and Bodo. We are eternally grateful to them, for their patience and sense of humour and willingness to repeat shots over and over again until they were just right. Many thanks to you both. Thanks also go to Gill for her support and type checking skills.

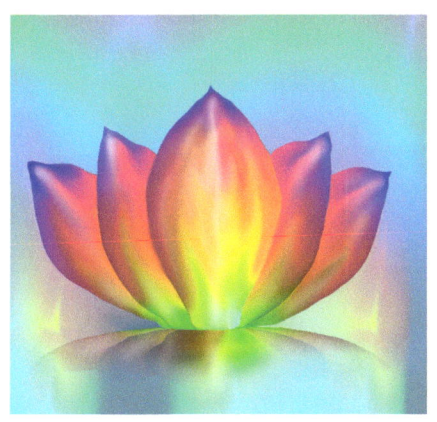

PREFACE

Welcome to this information packed book on romantic massage. Therapeutic touch is proven to be valuable, in fact essential, in maintaining emotional and physical well-being. Massage has been tried and tested over thousands of years. Physical touch strengthens emotional bonds and builds mutual trust - it can turn a failing relationship into a strong one - even help you to express your feelings or save a partnership. Now is your chance to try it.

At last, this is the book you have been waiting for. Learn about what oils to use, the underlying structure of your muscles and bones, when not to massage, and how and why you and your partner could benefit from each other's loving touch. Not only could you improve your relationship, you could help to soften and condition your skin, tone your muscles, reduce stress and lower your heart rate.

The book is packed with clear and tasteful photographs, showing sequences of strokes and positions. If 'a picture paints a thousand words' then this is a book you can't do without. You can dip into it to try a mini massage or why not work your way through - each chapter will give you graphic step by step instructions on a specific type of massage, from face massage to whole body massage. Try it and see, it doesn't matter how old you are, or how young your relationship is, we feel sure you will strengthen your relationship, improve your health .... and have some fun as well, as you get yourselves into some interesting positions!

1. TOUCHING MOMENTS

It has long been known that for humans and our distant cousins, the primates, physical touch and bonding are some of the most important contributors to a stable personality. Years ago, psychologists set up a somewhat distressing laboratory experiment, using baby monkeys, who were deprived of their mothers from an early age. They grew up emotionally disturbed and full of misery. We can relate this to humans. Unfortunately there are many insecure children and adults around who have been deprived of loving touch - the need is irrefutable.

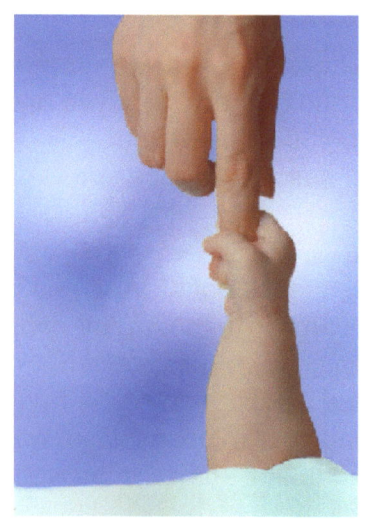

The human race is very complex, every creed and belief has an accepted code of conduct regarding touch - some forbid touching between the sexes, some forbid touching in public. Sometimes touching is used to 'test and sum up' each other, as in shaking hands, or giving a pat on the back.

However, touching and cuddling of babies is acceptable everywhere, it is a vital part of bonding, for parents, family, friends and, of course, the baby.

Gentle touch means "I love you, I care about you, you are important to me.' How sad it is that many adults never experience this type of touch - some don't even like touching and some never have the opportunity.

Many people get round this by having a pet dog or cat. Stroking the soft fur of a pet is known to calm and lower blood pressure. Many medical institutions allow dogs into hospital wards as this can be therapeutic to patients. Other people visit a therapist - there are many different kinds, most use touch as part of the treatment.

THERAPEUTIC TOUCH INDUCES RELAXATION

Therapeutic touch can be a wonderful way to facilitate both mental and physical relaxation. Massage therapy is becoming thoroughly acceptable these days. Until recently it was regarded as being a sexual practice, but before this, it was regularly used in hospitals to aid recovery from surgery and trauma. There is scientific evidence to prove this to be an effective treatment.

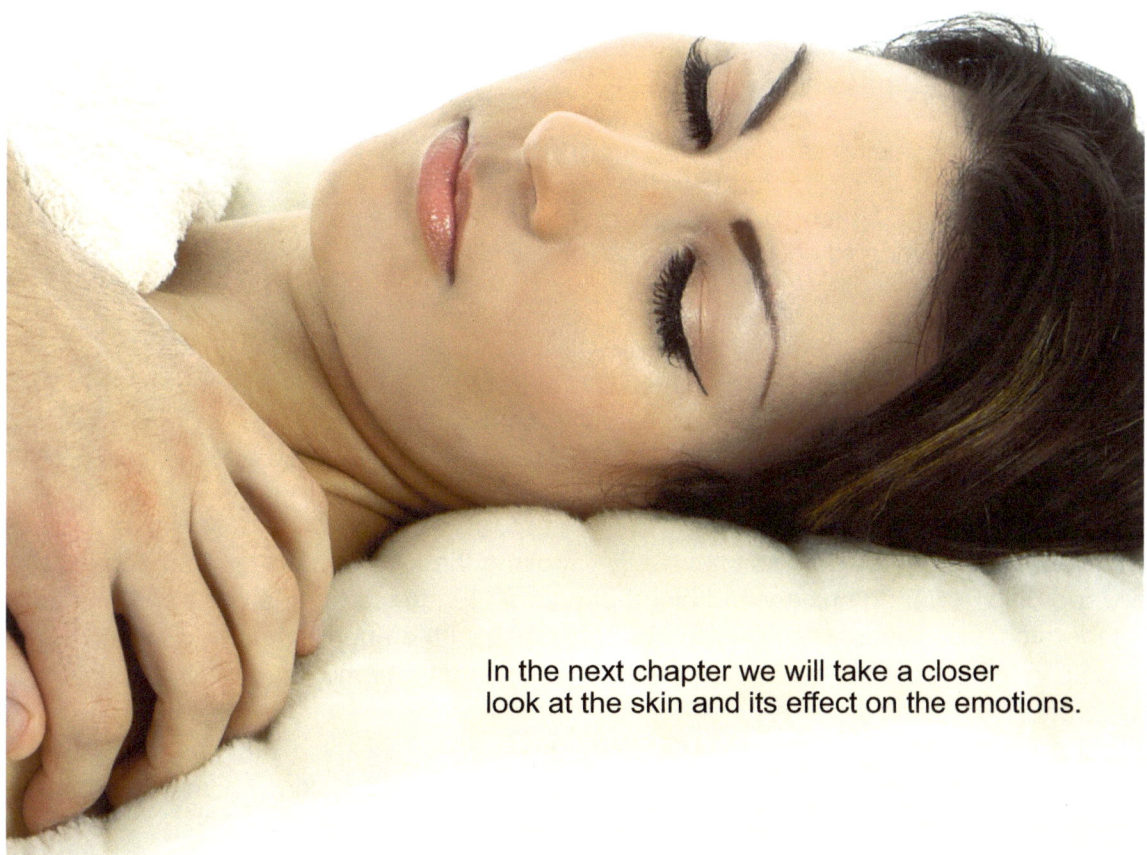

In the next chapter we will take a closer look at the skin and its effect on the emotions.

> YOUR SKIN COMPLETELY
> REPLACES ITSELF
> EVERY FIVE WEEKS

2. SKIN - A REMARKABLE ORGAN

The skin is the largest organ in the human body. Not only does it keep our insides in, it protects us from bacteria, helps our bodies to eliminate waste products, makes vitamin D (used in combination with calcium in the formation of bones, hair and teeth) regulates our body temperature, stores fat, protects our skeletons and gives us our shape.

It is constantly renewing itself, growing from the inside out. As the skin cells migrate to the surface they dry out and flatten, eventually forming a waterproof, waxy layer, protecting us against bacterial invaders.

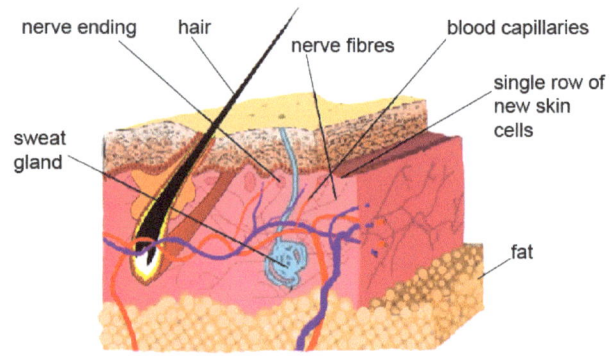

The texture and coloration of skin can indicate our state of health or our emotions. It is rich with nerve endings, especially in our fingertips, faces and feet. In fact the skin and nervous system arise from the same embryonic cells in the developing foetus.

It is no wonder that touch is so important - stroking the skin with a slow and gentle touch can be very soothing, lowering anxiety and blood pressure. Evidence for this has been monitored under laboratory conditions. We often see people blush with embarrassment, go white with shock, or come up in 'goose bumps' with fear - a strong indication that emotions affect the skin and its blood supply.

There is a huge network of tiny blood capillaries just under the skin, which gives light skinned people their pink colouring.

These blood capillaries are leaky, allowing nutritious fluids and oxygen to seep through their walls into the surrounding body tissues. The red blood cells (oxygen carrying haemoglobin) are

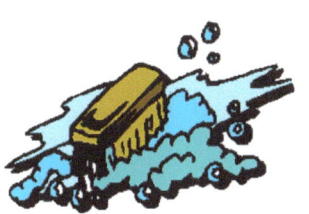

too big to get through the vessel walls but the oxygen detaches itself and slips through into the tissues, ready to help the cells to 'burn' the newly delivered fuel. This 'burning', amongst other things, produces the heat our bodies need to survive. The blood, now depleted of its oxygen, and carrying carbon dioxide, which it has gathered from the cells, turns blue and this can especially be seen in the veins in the wrists. This blue blood runs sluggishly back to the heart and lungs through the veins to gather more oxygen.

There is another network of lymphatic capillaries, which run very close to the blood capillaries and their job is to collect up the waste products from the tissue, and carry them away to be filtered out in the lymph nodes. If you liken blood capillaries to delivery vans, lymphatic capillaries are the refuse lorries, keeping the body clean and healthy. Knowing a little about these vital networks will help you to understand one of the main benefits of body massage, as gentle stroking, in the right direction can help to oxygenate the body's tissues and remove toxic substances.

3. TAKING CARE OF YOUR SKIN

The most important contributor to a healthy skin is a healthy diet and plenty of fresh clean water. After all, you are what you eat, skin is the largest organ in the body and is also an organ of elimination.

If you put junk food (and fluids) into your body, it will try to get rid of some of the waste products through your skin. Evidence for this can be seen in spotty skin, rough patches (especially on the backs of the arms and upper back) dandruff, skin infections and discoloration. You need water, at least a litre a day, to keep your skin moist and flexible (don't forget water is evaporating from your skin continuously, try wearing rubber gloves for an hour and they will soon be wet inside from evaporation). The caffeine in tea and coffee dehydrates the body by stimulating the kidneys, so keep consumption down to a minimum, and smoking causes yellowing and ageing.

A healthy diet consists of generous portions of fresh fruit and vegetables every day, as well as a good source of protein and high-fibre carbohydrates. This will give the body an adequate supply of vitamins and minerals and give you a lovely soft glowing skin. Adequate sleep is also vital, your body and mind need sleep time to rest and repair.

I can't stress enough, the importance of a healthy diet. If you are in a loving relationship, eating well is part of caring for each other, but you really should respect your body anyway.

I learnt this many years ago when I was going through a really bad patch in my life.

Being on my own and feeling thoroughly depressed, I stopped caring about myself and what I was eating. I would pick up cheap ready made meals from the supermarket, never bothering about fresh food. I only ate to survive and didn't feel I was worth bothering with. After a while my skin became rough and spotty, especially on the backs of my arms. Then I started feeling fuzzy headed, unable to concentrate, constantly tired and even more depressed. Then I developed an itchy, blistery skin rash which was diagnosed as chronic urticaria.

It took me three years to find out that I had a Candida overgrowth (Thrush). This yeast overgrowth in my gut was damaging it and making it leaky. This resulted in partially digested food particles getting into my bloodstream, causing an allergic reaction and an itchy blistery rash.

I eventually found a cure, by having an antibody blood test to find out which foods were causing the allergic reaction. I was then able to exclude these foods from my diet for three months. Gradually I introduced them again and improved my diet, learning to care for myself again.

As skin is the largest organ in the body, it is often used as a means of eliminating toxins. Massage is wonderful for encouraging the drainage and dispersal of waste products into the lymphatic system, as well as making you feel relaxed and better able to achieve restful sleep. Lavender is especially valuable as a sleep aid.

By all means moisturise your skin regularly but try to stick to natural vegetable oils - many commercial products contain a host of chemicals which could compromise your immune system.

As we age, the connective tissue just below the skin starts to lose its elasticity and then the underlying fat can bulge into the weakened structure, causing an 'orange peel' appearance. This is often more pronounced on the thighs and buttocks, as everything starts to sag a little with gravity. This orange peel skin is referred to as cellulite and applying creams to the skin will never totally restore the tone of the underlying skin structure.

Keeping skin flexible with oils and massage can help, especially if you have always looked after your skin, had a healthy diet and exercised regularly to keep your muscles firm. Stretch marks can be quite a problem, caused either by pregnancy or rapid weight gain. The connective tissue under the skin becomes overstretched and weak pockets develop, giving an uneven surface to the skin. Some people are more prone to these problems - if you can love yourself and not be made to feel inferior by beauty magazines and the media - you can live with little imperfections and still feel you are a beautiful person.

MASSAGE HELPS TO
CLEANSE THE BODY

4. ANYONE FOR A MASSAGE?

Body massage is a wonderful way of sharing quality time together. It is emotionally bonding, benefits your health and calms you down. However there are some circumstances where massage is unsuitable (contra-indications). Most of it is common sense, but I recently heard of a case where a lady with osteoporosis asked her friend for a back massage. The well-meaning friend was heavy handed and fractured a vertebra in her colleague's lower back, leaving her in awful pain. Don't massage if the following problems exist:

- Fragile or injured bones or joints, you could do more damage.

- Bruised or injured skin or underlying tissue.

- Ulcerated skin.

- Diabetics should be treated very carefully. Don't massage their toes if they have any problems such as cuts or bruises, ingrowing toenails, etc., as they could ulcerate and become gangrenous.

- Suspicious moles or skin cancer. Massage could spread dangerous cancerous cells into the bloodstream.

- Sunburnt skin.

- Any infectious or contagious conditions, or if you are unwell.

- Massage during pregnancy can be really special and comforting but don't use strong essential oils as some of them could induce early labour. Lavender is perfectly safe, you can use up to five drops in 10ml of carrier oil. Massage the abdomen with extra care and don't lie face down. Sitting, straddling a chair is good for a back massage.

PLEASE DON'T

- Drink alcohol, take drugs or smoke immediately after a massage, your body will be extra receptive to intoxicating or stimulating substances and you may be adversely affected.

- Use cheap synthetic essential oils. Many may smell inviting but they contain all sorts of chemicals, which will seep through the skin and get into the bloodstream.

- Massage for money. If you are not qualified and insured, and you cause injury, you could be sued for damage. You may do more harm than good.

You don't have to have a couch to perform a nice massage but if you take it seriously and want to make it part of your relationship, it would be a worthwhile investment.

It is important you don't strain your back reaching over your partner so you need to find somewhere that is comfortable for both of you. You can even massage lying side by side on the sofa or bed. I have been using massage as a healing therapy for years. I first discovered the comfort of massage when I was experiencing lower back pain, something which is very common in today's society.

Many osteopaths, chiropractors and physiotherapists use massage to loosen muscles before manipulation. If you or your partner have been having unexplained pain for any length of time you must see a medical practitioner before resorting to complementary therapies.

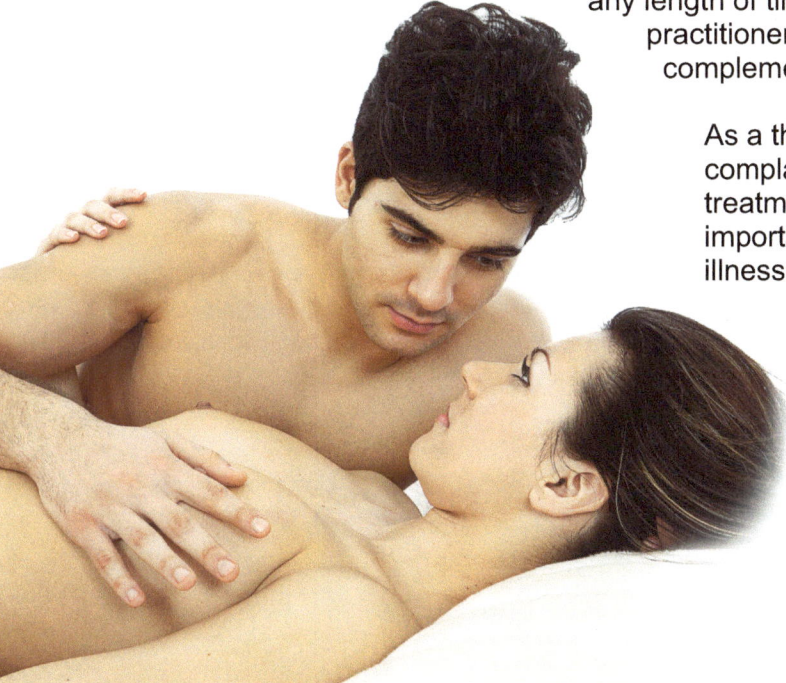

As a therapist I never diagnose medical complaints or prescribe drug treatments to my clients and it is important that you rule out serious illness before you treat each other.

There are many electrical aids available for you to use. If you don't have a willing partner you can   buy infrared lamps, vibratory massagers, heat pads and electric back massagers to help you to help yourself. Get yourself a vibratory massager with a long handle so you can reach awkward places.

Some gadgets have rotating 'fingers' which loosen tight muscles but they can be rather harsh and inhuman as well as being expensive. You put them behind you on a chair and lean on them. Whatever you decide try to test them first, some vibrate very fast and some hand held ones are a bit weak and ineffective. However nothing is a substitute for human touch. Having ruled out any reasons for not massaging, go ahead and prepare for a relaxing massage.

Aching muscles respond well, as you disperse irritating waste products from the tissue and increase blood supply, warming and nourishing the area. Get yourselves bottle of carrier oil (vegetable or sweet almond) oil, a small bottle of lavender oil, some towels, relaxing lighting and music and give each other some quality time.

Here we are demonstrating one of the electronic vibratory massagers. It has a long handle and sometimes I lie on my front on the bed and push it up and down my back to relieve muscular tension in my shoulders and upper back. It can be just as effective if used through clothing.

This particular massager has two speeds and heated infrared heads which are ideally spaced so you can run it either side of the spine. You need to be careful not to vibrate over bony tissue such as the vertebrae, shoulder blades or shins. I don't use it near the head area (brain) or vital organs such as the heart as it is quite strong and could cause problems. Using a towel cushions the body just enough and helps to keep you warm.

If you have any peripheral nerve damage (tingling, numbness or pain in your fingers or toes) as in a disc injury, use the vibrator with care as it can irritate tetchy nerves. Diabetes can also cause diminished feeling in the hands and feet. Please proceed with caution. As stated earlier, diabetics are prone to serious foot problems if skin or blood vessels are damaged.

MASSAGE IS EMOTIONALLY BONDING

5. GETTING STARTED

Before you start make sure that the room is warm, draught free, private, undisturbed and comfortable. You may wish to spread a large bath towel on the bed or even work on the living room floor. Make sure the area is soft and padded with some cushions though, or some of the firmer strokes may cause discomfort.

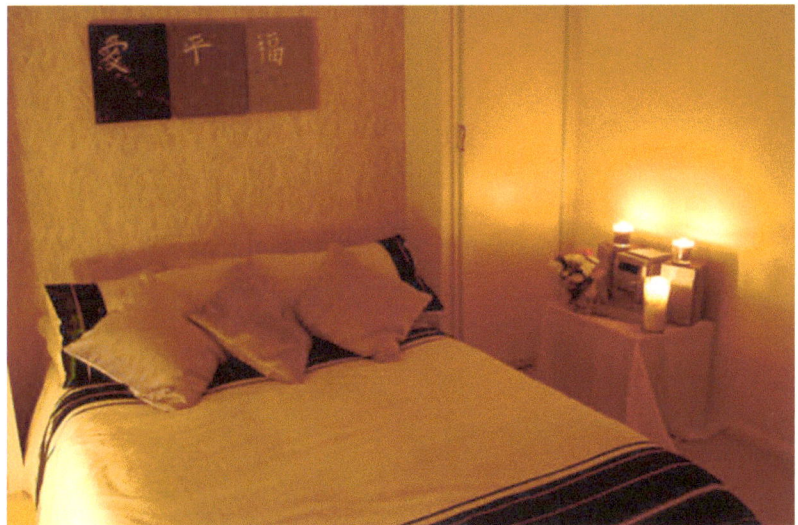

You may wish to have a warm bath or shower first. It is nice to feel warm and clean before a massage and if you use oils you may wish to shower off the excess afterwards.

Body massage is always best on a naked body. This allows the 'therapist' to perform long sweeping strokes along the body without worrying about underwear. If your partner is shy, turn down the lighting. He or she could just keep basic underwear on but this may get oily. Cover your partner with a large towel or or two and wrap them up if they are chilly and just concentrate on one part of the body at a time.

You will need oils, creams or talcum powder, a couple of large towels, a small cushion (wrapped in an old pillow case), a saucer for the oil/lotion, some relaxing music, and a dressing gown or towel for the therapist (unless you wish to do the massage without clothes). You could use couch roll or some old, clean sheeting, to protect your towels and bed. I use a microwavable plate warmer to keep the saucer of oil warm, but you could also use a wheat bag.

I also use incense to make the room smell deliciously oriental. If possible dim the lighting, close the curtains and have a portable heater if the temperature is cool - even if you, the therapist, gets warm, your partner may well feel chilly, especially if you use a lotion, which evaporates from the body. I use an electric fan heater which warms the room up quickly and is easy to turn on and off.

You oould, of course, perform massage in the bath, space permitting. Use a nice liquid soap and massage the arms, chest and tummy. Use shampoo as a lubricant for the head and give a nice stimulating head massage. Or how about giving your partner a lovely back, head and neck massage in the shower? (using a non-slip mat). If you have sensitive skin you can use an emollient body lo such as E45 cream.

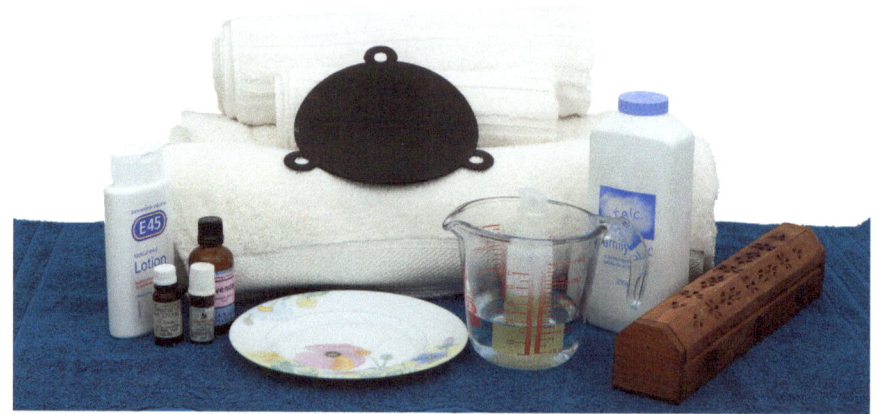

ESSENTIAL OILS MAY SOOTHE INFLAMMATION, ACT AS AN ANTISEPTIC, HELP DULL PAIN AND STIMULATE DIGESTION

6. ESSENTIAL OILS TO AFFECT THE EMOTIONS

Essential oils are produced by plants, which mainly grow in hot climates. They often contain a complex cocktail of chemicals, designed to protect the plants from predators and evaporation, in the heat of the sun. They are often volatile, that is they atomise easily and escape into the air. Well-known essential oils are lavender, rosemary and cedar wood. These natural essences are extensively used in household products, their attractive scents make our homes smell nice.

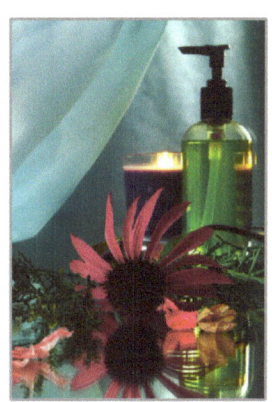

The art of Aromatherapy is the practice of using essential oils to affect or change your mood. Oils are said to have uplifting or calming effects. They are categorized into 'high, mid and low notes'. Lemon oil is typically uplifting, while lavender can help you to relax.

Aromatherapists will establish with careful questions what your emotional needs are, and then mix a cocktail of essences into a base (carrier) oil to get the desired effect. Later on we will discuss some typical emotional needs within a relationship, such as lack of communication, drifting apart etc. and suggest some oils to bring about a balance.

How can these oils change your mood? Essential oils can easily get into the body during massage because the skin is semi-permeable, that is, there are tiny spaces between the skin cells through which the oils enter. They permeate into the layer of natural fat under the skin and are then absorbed into the blood and lymph. They are carried in tiny quantities to receptors in the brain. These receptors are designed to receive natural

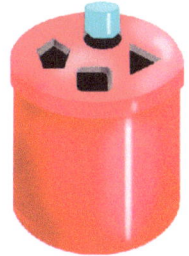

chemicals, such as endorphins, which have a specific shape, a bit like childrens' shape sorters. Molecules from essential oils also fit some of the receptors, causing a beneficial change of mood. The membranes in the nose also allow the atomised oils into the body. Some oils such as Clary sage can make you feel quite 'heady'.

Some essential oils are very potent and can burn the skin. NEVER apply these oils neat to the skin, even tea tree oil, which can irritate some skins and cause dermatitis. Store your oils in a dark glass bottle, preferably in a cool place such as a fridge, to keep them fresh and effective

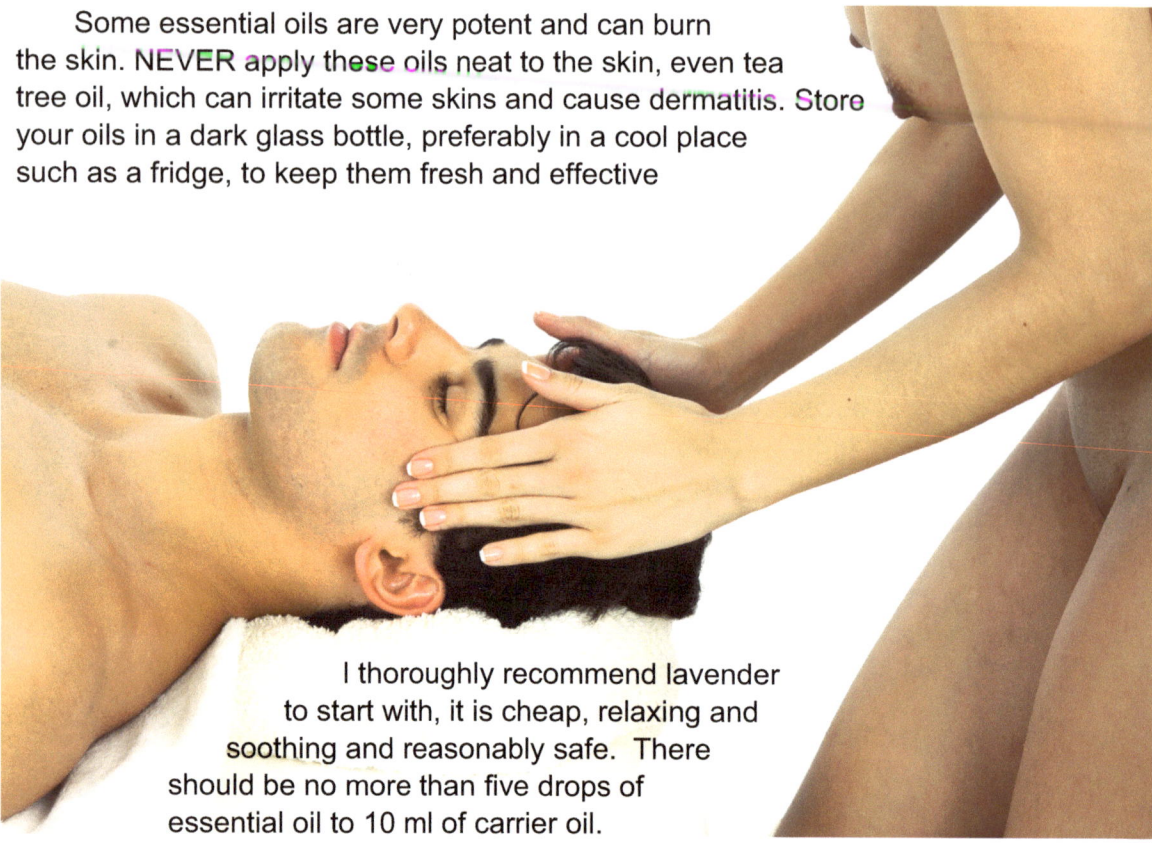

I thoroughly recommend lavender to start with, it is cheap, relaxing and soothing and reasonably safe. There should be no more than five drops of essential oil to 10 ml of carrier oil.

Carrier oils need to be fresh and not rancid. You can use sweet almond oil (unless allergic to nuts), pure cooking oils such as corn oil, grape-seed or olive oil, rice bran oil, coconut oil or even baby creams and lotions. If in doubt, use emollient cream or E45 cream if you have eczema, dermatitis or other skin problems. You can buy ready mixed massage oils but many contain chemicals and synthetic perfumes which are not ideal as these will be absorbed into your body.

If you don't like getting messy you can use talcum powder, but this may dry the skin. You can even mix a little almond oil with baby lotion and lavender oil for a delightful massage. The important thing is to have enough slip and slide to avoid friction and soreness. Vegetable oils stay slippery for a long time and baby lotions tend to soak in quicker. Oil can stain clothing if not washed off immediately, so clean off any excess on the skin before getting dressed and wash towels as soon as possible after use. I find that vegetable oils will leave a yellow stain on towels and bedding if you don't wash them regularly. Leave the oil on the skin for as long as possible as it is very beneficial and nourishing, helping to keep your skin soft and supple.

Before you start ensure your nails are short, to avoid scratching. If your hands are rough, rub them over with a pumice stone (in soapy water) to remove the dead skin. You should always wash your hands first anyway, ensuring they are warm.

MASSAGE CAN RELIEVE PAIN
BY AIDING NATURAL HEALING
IN THE BODY'S TISSUES.

7. BASIC MASSAGE TECHNIQUES

Effleurage Long, slow strokes, using the palms of both hands in wide sweeping movements. It spreads the oil evenly over the skin and is very soothing.

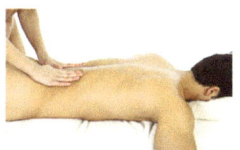 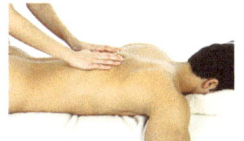 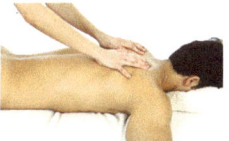

Kneading As its name implies, is a deep movement used on large areas of soft tissue such as the upper back and buttocks. It helps to eliminate waste products from the body, to breakdown fatty tissue, and aid decongestion.

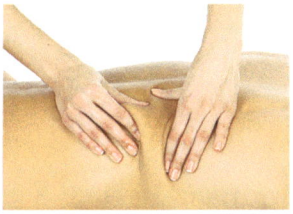

Petrissage 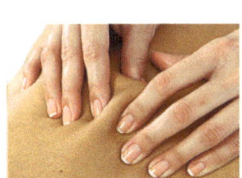 Concentrated kneading, using small, localised movements. It is used on areas of tissue with bone underneath, such as shoulder blades. It helps to soothe and tone muscle fibres. It also encourages the dispersal of waste products in the skin.

Firm pressure with the fingertips, often either side of the spine. The fingers are vibrated rapidly from side to side as they are pushed along the underlying muscle fibres - a good technique for releasing tension along both sides of the spine.

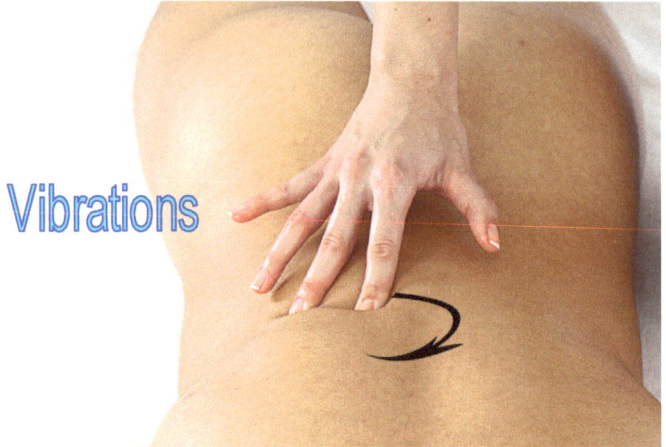
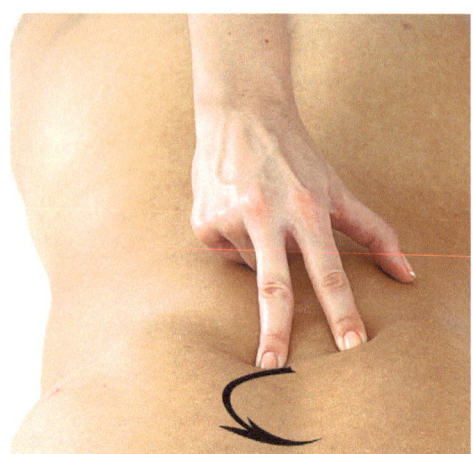

Vibrations

Often used together, cupping creates a vacuum to draw more blood to the surface. Hacking is done by rapidly hitting the tissue with the outer edge of the hands. This is best used where there is muscular tension, for example in the buttocks, shoulder, back and thighs.

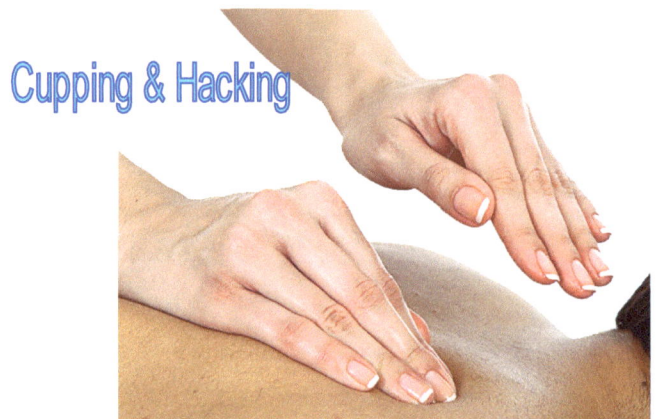
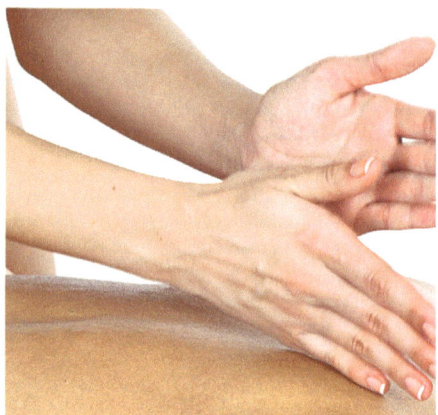

Cupping & Hacking

Tapotement

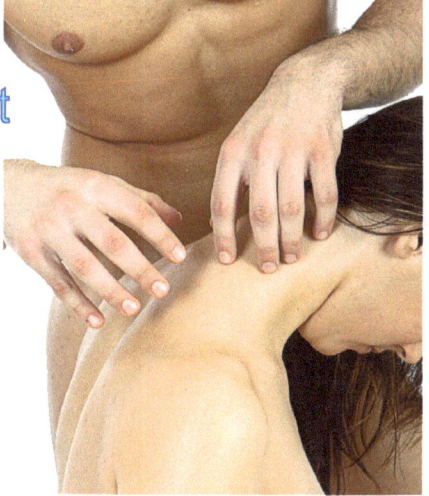

A tapping movement, using the fingers and alternate hands, which stimulates the circulatory system

Knuckling

Making a fist and using the knuckles to knead the tissue. This is good on the upper back and shoulders

Wringing

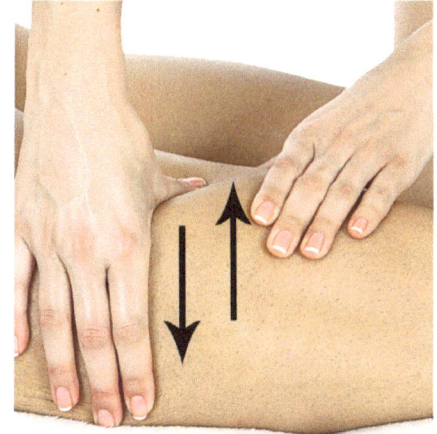
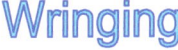

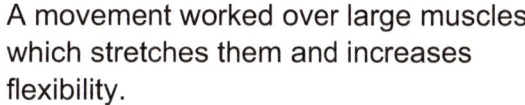

A movement worked over large muscles which stretches them and increases flexibility.

ONE SQUARE CENTIMETRE OF MUSCLE HAS UP
TO ONE MILLION FIBRES, EACH OF
WHICH IS COMMANDED BY A
NERVE TO MAKE IT CONTRACT

8. WHOLE BODY MASSAGE

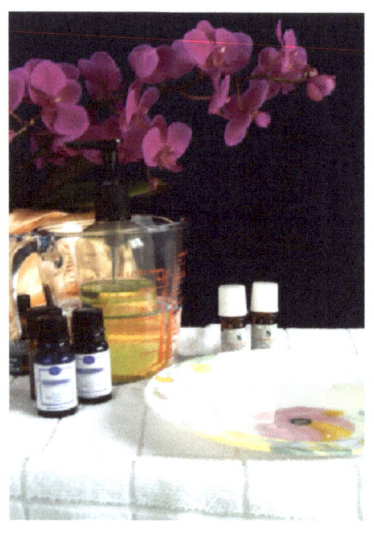

Pour some massage oil into the saucer so you can dip the palm of your hands into it. You could use a bottle but you will have to keep stopping to pick it up to squeeze more oil out, and this interrupts the flow of the treatment. You can warm the oil by leaving the bottle in a jug of hot water for 5 minutes or you could rest the saucer of massage mixture on a hot wheat bag or microwavable plate warmer to keep it warm throughout the session. Sometimes, as a therapist, I mix some E45 cream with the oil so it rubs in quicker and doesn't leave my client's skin too oily. This could stain their clothes, on their way home. Also I usually rub the excess off with a soft towel, for the same reason.

Make sure your partner is comfortable and warm. Cover him or her with a warm towel if the temperature is a bit chilly, placing the pillow under the head, lying face up. A heat pad on the couch, or a warm wheat bag will help to warm up stiff muscles in the back. Remove all jewellery and put on some soft relaxing music. (My 'Inner Harmony' CD is ideal)

Here you can see a diagram of the musculature of the arm and why it is important to massage along the fibres to disperse waste products towards the lymph nodes under the arm. Uncover one arm at a time and apply the oil, moving your hands slowly and rhythmically along the muscles.

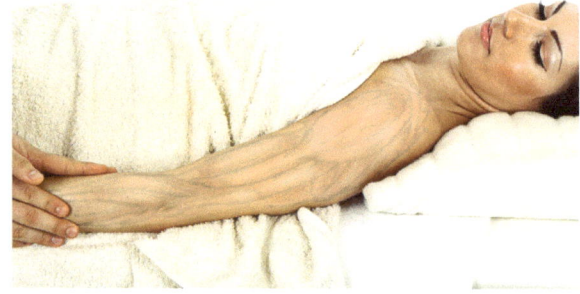

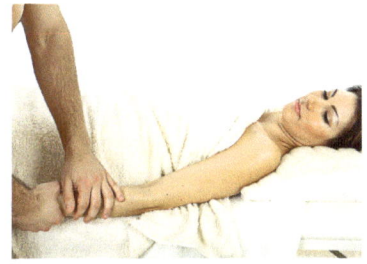 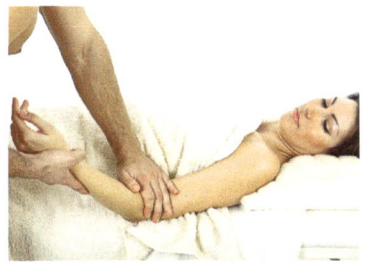 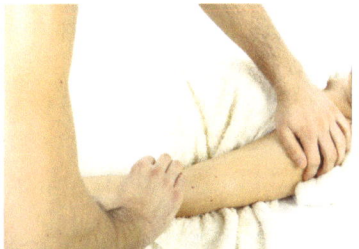

Starting at the wrist, push firmly along the arm, one hand over the other and keeping in constant contact. This rhythmic flowing motion helps to move waste products towards the heart, liver and kidneys, and thence out of the body. Use nice firm strokes but don't bruise or hurt. Flimsy strokes can by irritating and you may need to practice to get the pressure right. Make sure you give each other feed-back on how things are going.

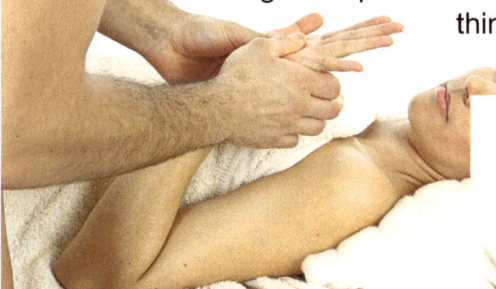 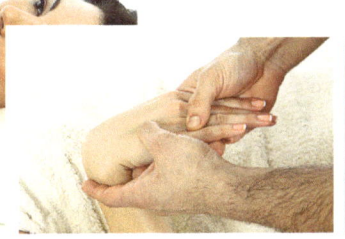 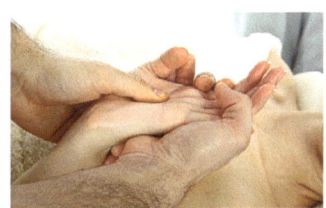

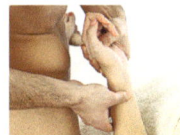 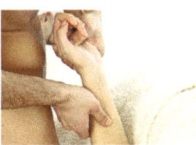 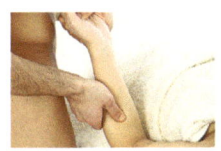

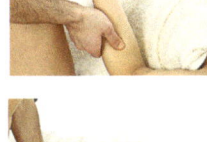

Work your way along the muscles of the arm, pushing upwards towards the lymph nodes in the armpits.

Use plenty of lubricant and keep the movements slow and rhythmic.

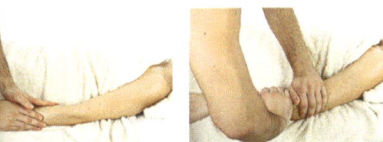 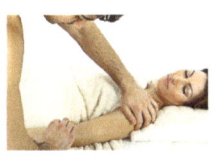

If the skin is rough or spotty here, it could indicate a need for a better, more balanced diet. If you continually eat processed or junk food your body will try to eliminate waste products through your skin. Ask your partner to raise their arm and rest their hand on your chest, using gravity to drain stale blood towards the lymph nodes in the armpit.

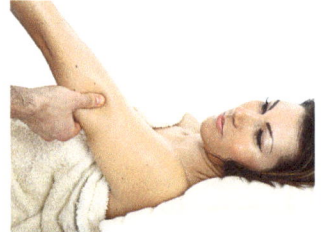 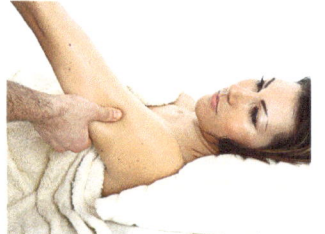 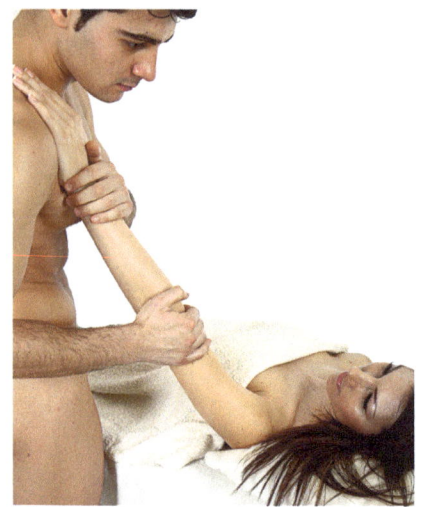

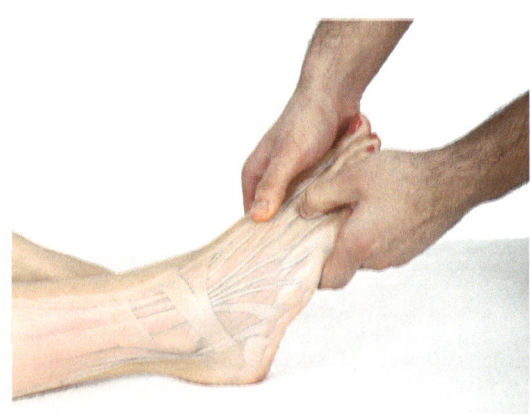

Now we move to the feet and legs. The picture on the left shows the position of the tendons. If your partner is chilly tuck the arms back under cover before starting on the fronts of the legs, one at a time. Feet can be very sensitive so make sure you get feedback from your partner.

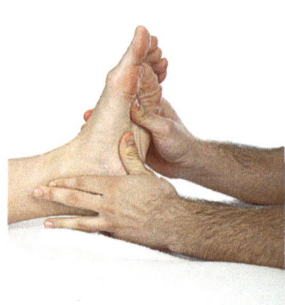

As long as your partner isn't too ticklish use a firm pressure to work your thumbs across the sole of the foot, round the toes and over the arch of the foot.

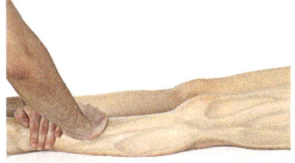 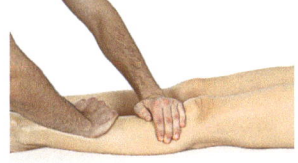 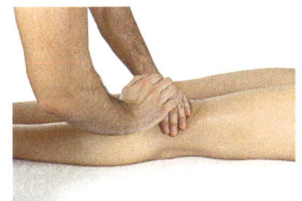 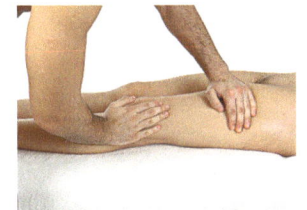

Go carefully over bony areas and, like the arms, push up, along the muscles (shown above) towards the groin. There are lymph nodes at the back of the knee and in the groin, so bear this in mind as you carefully guide the lymphatic fluid in that direction.

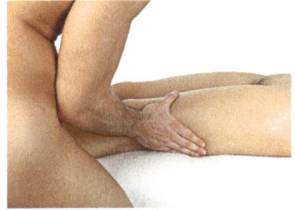 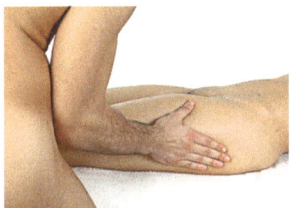 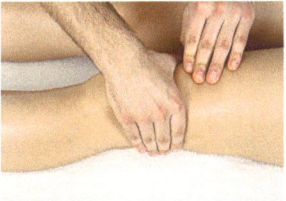 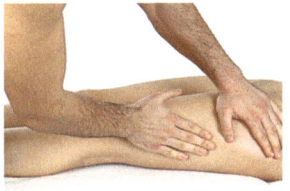

In the privacy of your home it is fine to gently massage the erogenous zones but don't stop your massage routine, intimacy can come later. If your partner is naked, you can massage the outside of the upper legs and over the hip joints, up to the waist. There are a variety of strokes you can use and we will demonstrate them later. Don't be alarmed if the skin reddens, this is a good sign. Enjoy the texture and smoothness of your partner's skin as you follow the routine.

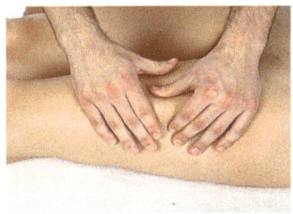 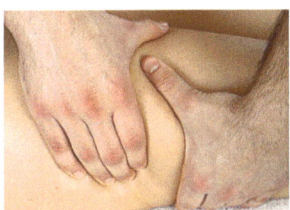 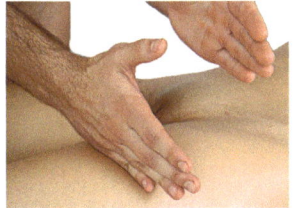 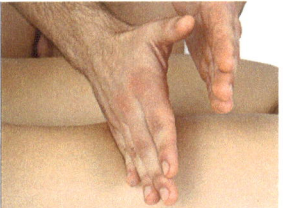

Here our models are demonstrating kneading, wringing and hacking on the tops of the legs.

Next you can massage the trunk. Again, being naked is ideal and massaging around the rib cage and breast tissue is very beneficial. The incidence of breast problems, including cancer, is far higher in the developed world and there is evidence that the wearing of tight bras can restrict the flow of lymph, causing a build up of waste products and toxins. It is also a good idea to check for suspicious lumps or bumps, both in male and female breast tissue. Massaging can be very erotic for both men and women, so enjoy the experience.

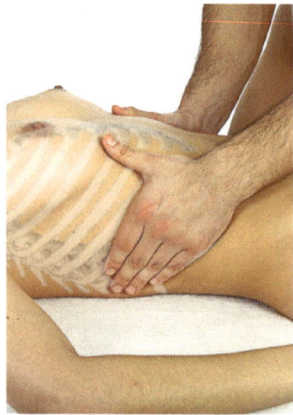

Massage the rib cage first, (shown here) following the direction of the ribs from front to back. If your female partner has tender breasts use gentle slow movements, moving around the breasts in a circular motion.

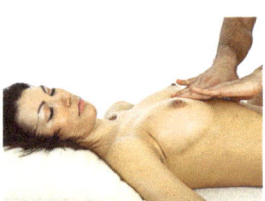 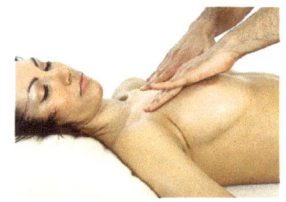 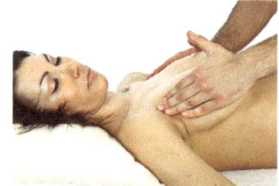

Massaging the chest area is so beneficial and comforting too. If you sit at a computer all day or have a sedentary job, the muscles around the rib cage, collar bones and shoulders don't get much exercise. Stiffness can develop over the rib cage as we age, and this encourages shallow breathing. This in turn can cause acidity in the blood, an unhealthy condition which leaves us open to illness and diseases. Take some deep breaths during the massage to oxygenate the body and enhance relaxation.

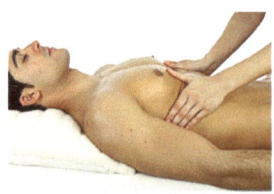 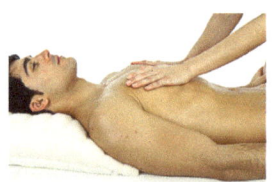 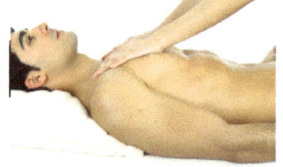 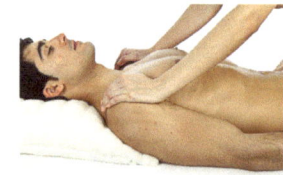

Then move from the centre of the chest across the collar bones, towards the shoulders and lymph nodes under the arm.

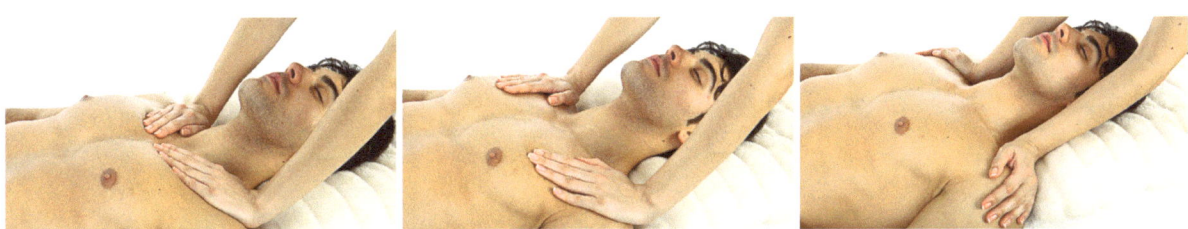

Give the shoulders a thorough massage as this is where there is often a lot of tension and potential muscular problems. It is beneficial to work along the edge of the rib cage. Starting at the base of the breast bone (sternum) work your well oiled fingers, with firm strokes, along the bottom edge of the rib cage. The ribs' intercostal muscles work constantly to make you breathe, and giving them a work-over keeps them supple.

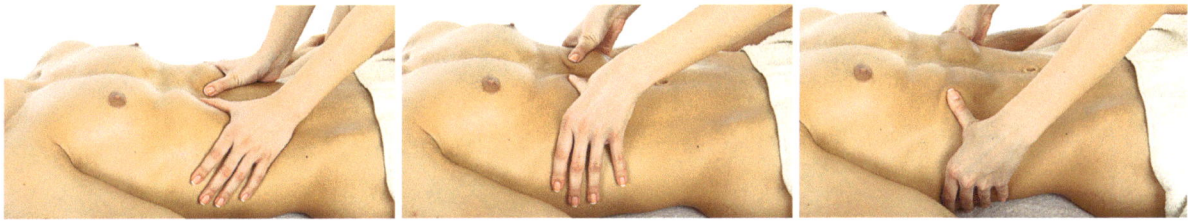

Lastly, you can massage the abdomen. If your female partner is pregnant use plenty of oil and gently massage over and around the developing baby. This is very beneficial for the baby, who will enjoy the therapeutic touch. It is also beneficial to its mother's slowly stretching skin.

The digestive tract (all 20 feet of it!) is the main occupant of the abdomen. The small intestine is tightly packed inside, leading into the colon. This is the final stage of digestion and faecal matter moves through the colon in a clockwise direction and down to the rectum and anus, ready for elimination.

Move your hands slowly and firmly in a clockwise direction, starting above the right hip as shown. Sweep right, across the naval and down towards the left hip. Here we see the position of the colon.

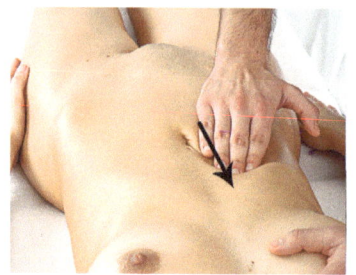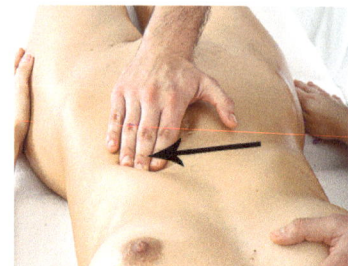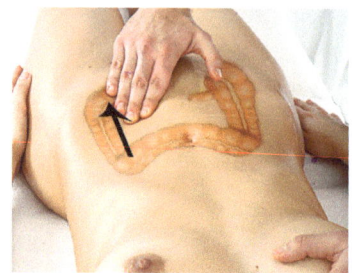

Repeat this four or five times, this will encourage the faeces to move and speed up elimination. Don't press too hard, especially if there is trapped wind, as it can be very uncomfortable

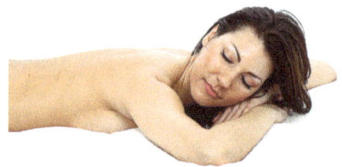 It is now time to turn over. Gently help your partner, who should be feeling very relaxed and floppy

If you are working on the floor or the bed, you could straddle your partner so you are not twisting your spine

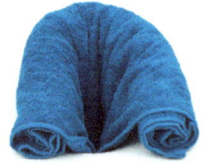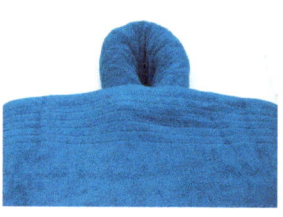

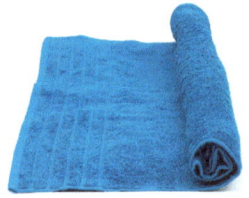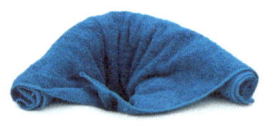

If you have a couch with a face hole, roll up a small bath towel, leaving about 30cm to tuck into the hole. Curve it round, tuck neatly into the hole and place another towel over the ends to stop it opening up. This makes a comfortable padding for your partner's face..

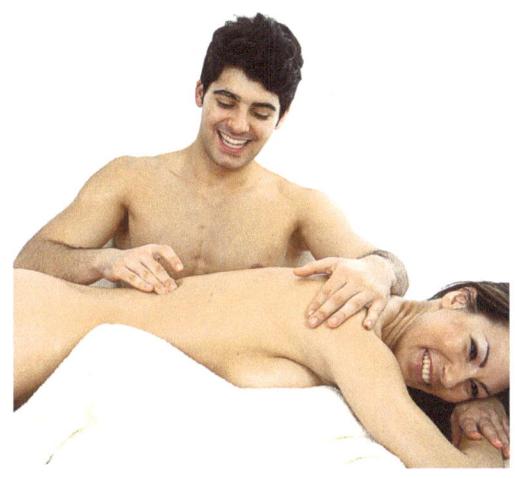

Or you could sit down, place some cushions on your lap and have your partner lie across your lap

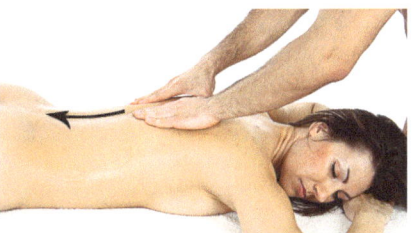

If your partner has to turn their head to the right or left, get them to change regularly as they could overstretch the neck muscles. Standing at your partner's head end and starting at the shoulders, push firmly down either side of the spine to the top of the pelvis.

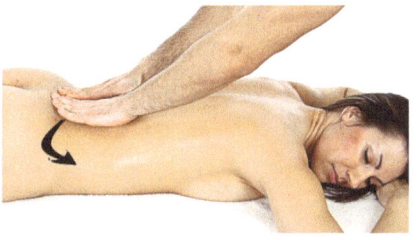

Sweep your hands firmly down over the top of the pelvis and then pull them up towards you, either side of the body, to the shoulders, in a circular movement. Repeat this several times. This will help to stretch the vertebrae apart, open up the small of the back, and stretch the inter-costal muscles of the rib cage.

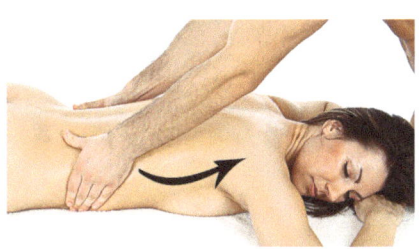

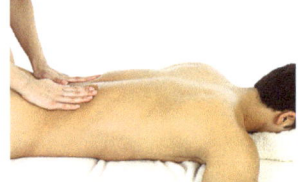 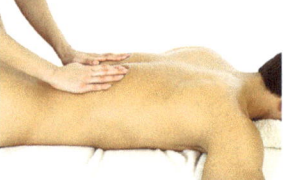 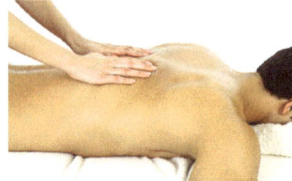 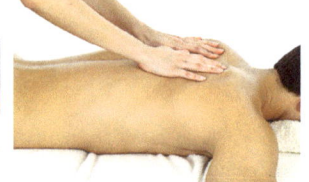

Push firmly along the spine to ease the compression between the vertebrae

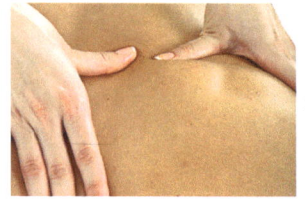

Feel for knots over shoulder blades

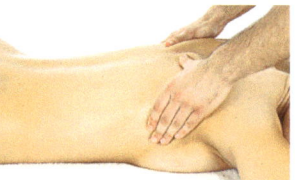

Use long sweeping movements to increase circulation

Soften knotty tissue with your knuckles

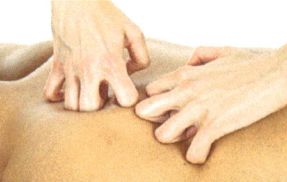

Squeeze and knead the muscles over the shoulders

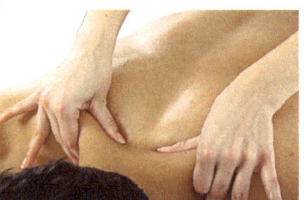

Don't worry if the skin reddens (erythema), this is an indication that blood flow is increasing, bringing nutrients to the skin and muscles and eliminating a build up of waste products from the tissues.

Our muscles are arranged in layers and bundles and are designed to slide against each other. However, stress, lack of exercise, poor posture, poor diet, insufficient water intake and restrictive clothing stops waste products from being effectively removed and muscles become less elastic and more sticky. A build-up of waste products in the tissue causes acidity, which in turn irritates local nerves and causes pain.

Run your hands in long sweeps from the waist, down the buttocks to the thighs. Be careful not to pull the buttocks apart as this can damage the delicate skin between them.

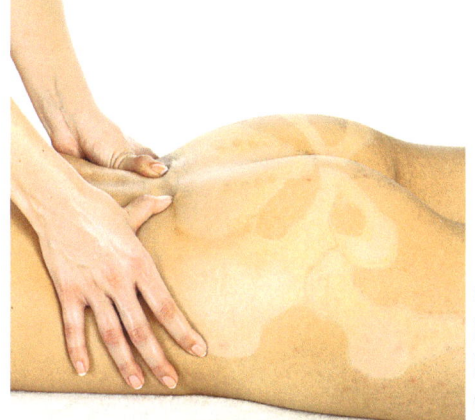
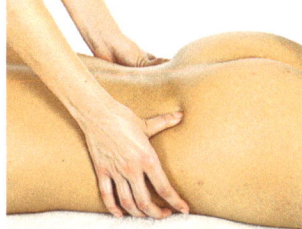
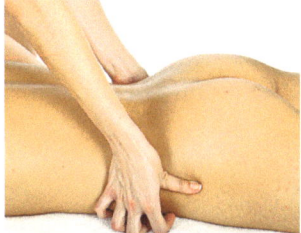

Work thoroughly over the rim of the pelvic girdle (shown here) and buttocks, pushing down from the lower back to the hip and kneading with your fingers and knuckles. This area will often feel tender as it is subject to wear and tear.

In women, the pelvis needs to expand during childbirth, and there should be a certain amount of flexibility of this area. Regularly massaging and manipulating the sacroiliac joint can help to save the lower spine from back injury.

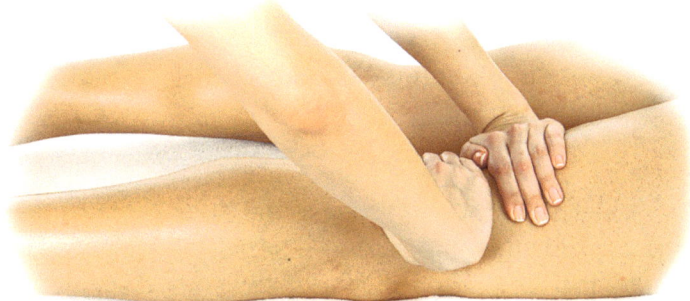

Next we come to the backs of the legs. Unless the room is very warm, cover up the back with a towel and, starting with the ankles, spread the oil, working your way up the backs of the legs and thighs. If there are varicose veins don't press hard over this area as it can make them worse. Push all the stale blood in the leg veins up towards the body   and lymph nodes, paying particular attention to the upper thighs.

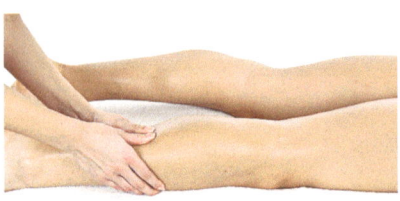 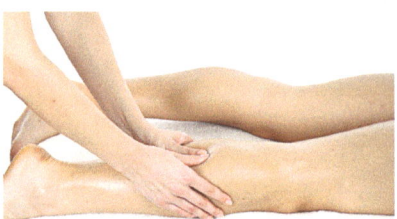 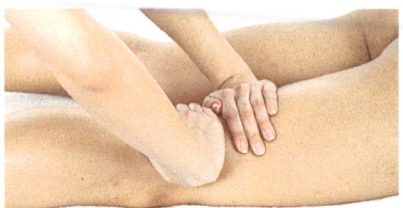

The last part of your massage session should be concentrated on the neck and shoulders. We all bear our emotions in these areas. No wonder we suffer from headaches and pains in the shoulders.

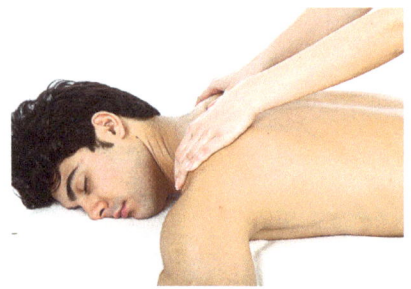 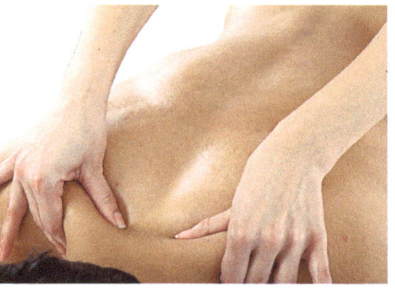 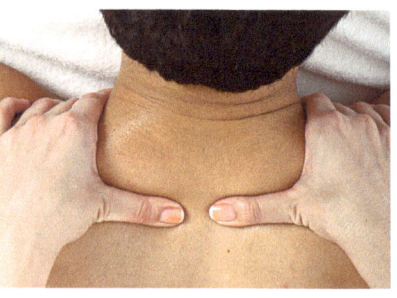

Use firm strokes, moving from the shoulders to the neck

Knead and squeeze the shoulder muscles

Press either side of the spine and along the base of the skull

You can feel the bundles of fibres in the huge trapezius muscle, which is attached to either side of the spine just above the waistline and stretches up the back in a triangular shape. It then runs either side of the neck and across the top of the shoulders. This muscle pulls the head and shoulders back and is prone to aches and pains caused by stress and lack of exercise.

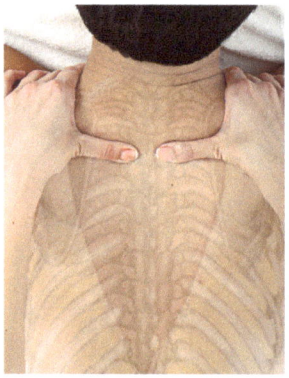

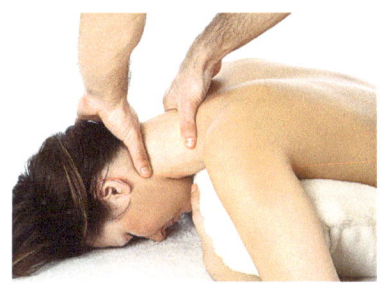

Work on the knotty fibres. Work your fingers up either side of the cervical spine up to the base of the skull.

Work along the bottom ridge of the skull, fingering your way along and pressing as you go.

Again this may feel tender as this area tightens up when we are stressed. Your loving strokes will do so much to make your partner feel relaxed, so make the most of it.

You can signal the end of your massage with a tender kiss or cuddle. Allow your partner a minute or two to 'surface' from a state of bliss.

It is important that you offer your partner a long cool drink of water. Massage increases the movement of lymph through the body, draining the fluids via the heart into the kidneys. There is now space for fresh water - an essential component of a healthy body.

Like a clean sponge, the body will readily soak up whatever you put into it, so avoid toxins such as alcohol, drugs, caffeine, cigarettes etc. You may also both feel relaxed but tired and at the end of your romantic day, you should enjoy a good night's sleep.

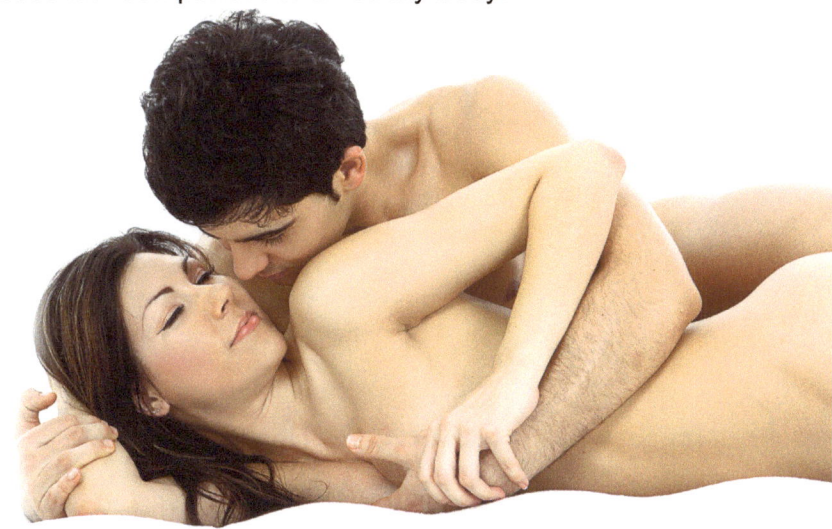

> REGULAR MASSAGE GIVES MUSCLES
> INCREASED FLEXIBILITY AND RANGE
> OF MOVEMENT

9. MINI MASSAGES -
INDIAN HEAD MASSAGE

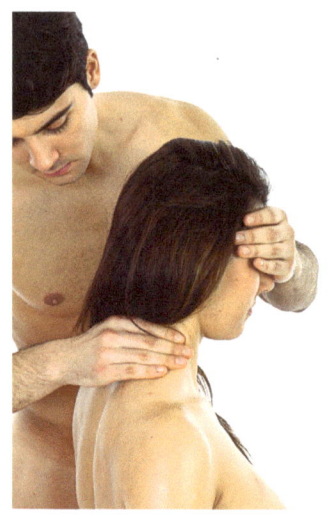

This form of head and shoulder massage has been handed down for generations and is regularly practised in India. Whole families will be involved, the youngsters will massage the grandparents, the husbands will treat the wives. They use different oils for different seasons, some are warming and invigorating, some are soothing and cooling.

Regular oiling of the hair and scalp ensures healthy hair and supple skin but Indian Head Massage can be used without it, the act of manipulating the scalp is very beneficial.

Head massage can be performed any time and does not need as much preparation as body massage. As long as the room is peaceful and you are not interrupted, you can give each other a lovely massage whilst listening to your favourite music.

As with body massage, qualified therapists use a series of strokes and a set routine for Indian Head Massage. This ensures that the client derives maximum benefit from their treatment in the allotted time. However you can experiment with the strokes we have demonstrated in the photographs and set your own routine. Moving the scalp around over the skull is very beneficial and enjoyable. Massaging the neck and shoulders is also a wonderful way of sharing your caring feelings for your partner

Starting your massage routine

If you are the receiver, find somewhere comfortable to sit, in a relaxing environment. Have some lovely soothing music nearby - a few scented candles would also be nice. The 'therapist' can either stand behind or sit on a higher level. For example one could sit on the settee while the other nestles on a cushion on the floor, between their legs. Or one could sit in a chair with their partner standing behind.

Don't use a high backed seat or you won't be able to massage around the shoulder blades. Swiveling chairs on wheels are no good either as you can't apply enough pressure without the chair moving. A low stool would be ideal, or you could sit on the floor. The beauty of Indian Head Massage is that it can also be done fully clothed, so it can be spontaneous and unplanned.

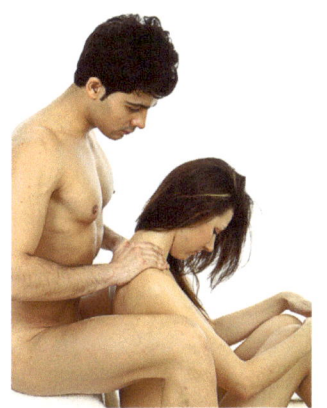

We will call our couple James and Sarah. Sarah is seated between James' knees on the floor while James tenderly places his hands on Sarah's shoulders and listens to her breathing.

Soon James is able to synchronise his breathing with Sarah's, as her shoulders rise and fall with each breath.

James now applies some oil to Sarah's scalp. They are using sweet almond oil and James has put a few drops of cedarwood in for its calming and relaxing qualities. He gently works the oil into the scalp and roots of the hair. It isn't obligatory to use oil but there are many benefits, so give it a try some time.

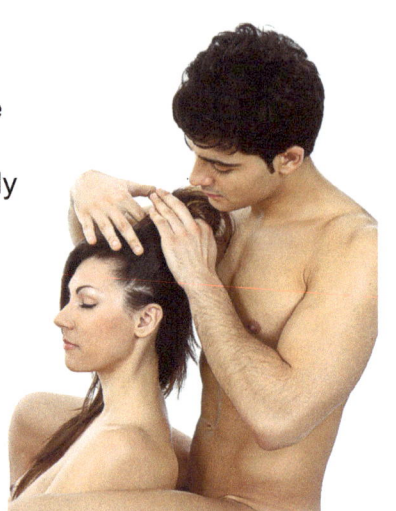

Steadying her head with his left hand he briskly rubs the right side of Sarah's head, just in front of her ear, moving round to behind the ear, in a 'windscreen wiper' motion. He repeats this a few times on one side and does the same on the other. This stimulates the scalp and is surprisingly pleasant.

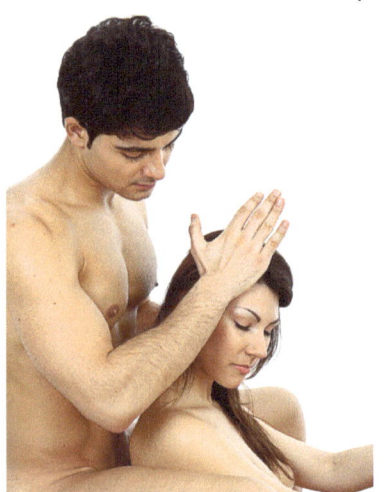 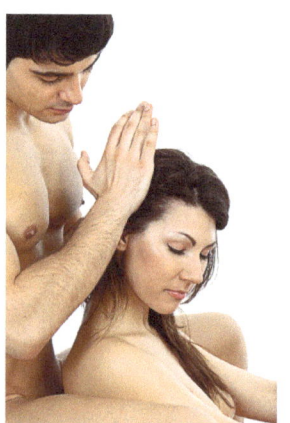 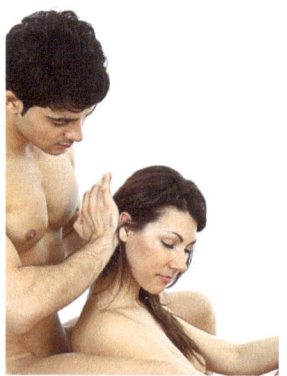

Leave the oil on the hair for a while before shampooing it off. It nourishes the hair, softens it, gives it elasticity and conditions the skin on the scalp.

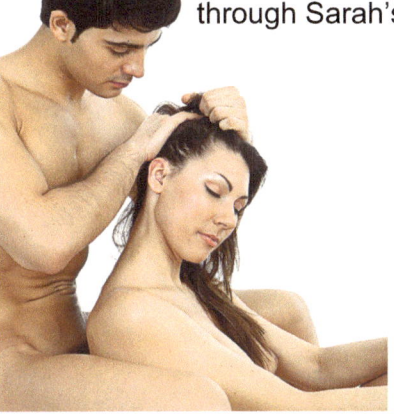 James uses his fingertips to slowly and rhythmically move the scalp around over the underlying skull - a bit like applying shampoo. He then works the oil through Sarah's hair, from roots to tips, a few strands at a time.

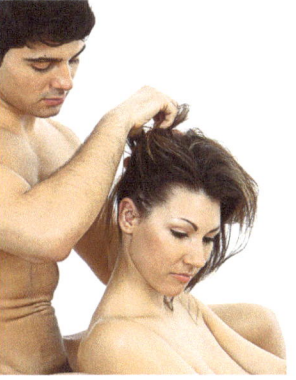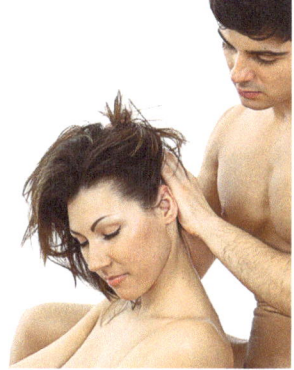

He gently tugs the locks of hair, stimulating the scalp and increasing the blood flow. Sarah enjoys it as James then briskly rubs her scalp all over, stimulating the roots of the hair and blood supply to the skin.

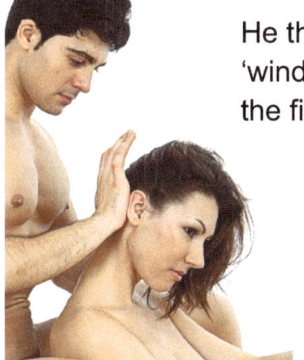 He then rubs the base of her skull, in a 'windscreen wiper' movement, similar to the first movement of the session

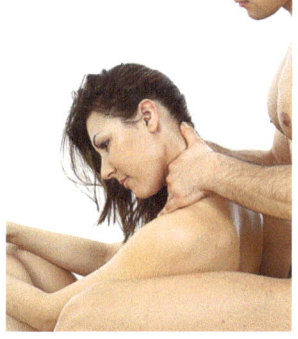

Then, working his way along the base of her skull with his fingertips, he presses gently from the back of one ear from one side to the other.

This area is often sore and tension headaches can arise from here.

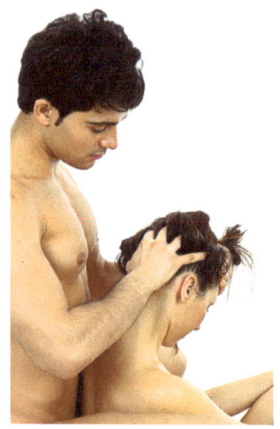

James finishes the head massage with a series of deep rubbing movements, moving the scalp around and lubricating the hair. He places one hand over Sarah's forehead and one at the back of the head. He squeezes his hands together as he pushes upwards towards the crown. This is a great movement for releasing all the tension in the scalp muscles.

James then puts his right hand at the back of his partner's neck, with the other hand on her forehead. He asks Sarah to relax as he rocks her head back a few times, stretching the neck muscles in preparation for a neck massage.

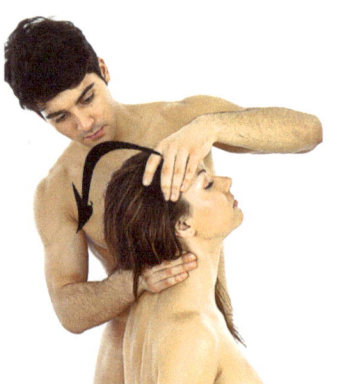
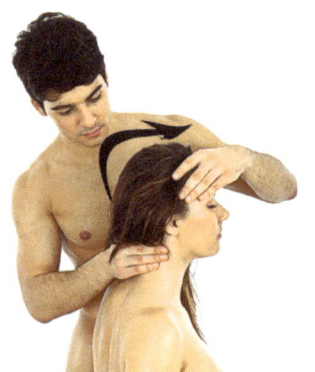
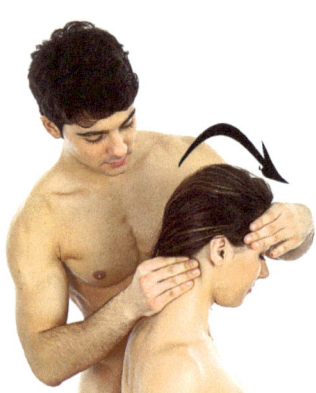

His hands are still well oiled. If you are not using oil in your massage, you may wish to apply a little baby lotion at this stage.

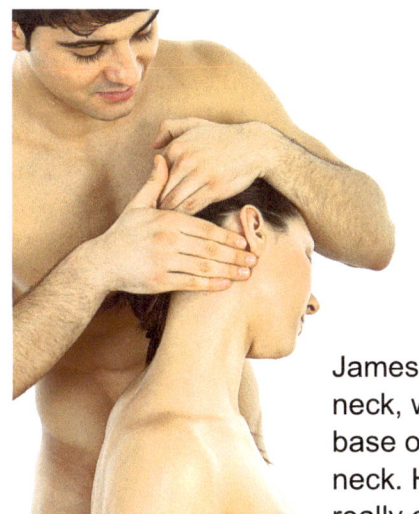

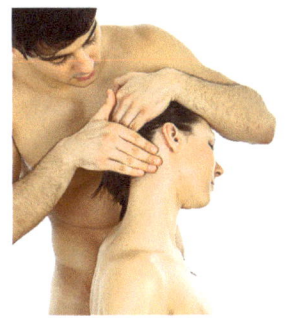

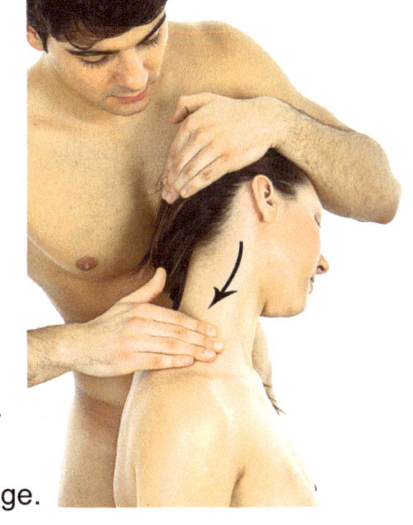

James firmly massages Sarah's neck, working his way from the base of her skull to the nape of her neck. He takes his time as Sarah really enjoys this part of the massage.

It is important to have well oiled hands here, as this skin is quite delicate. James steadies Sarah's head with his left arm and massages the right side of her neck, down to her shoulder. He then steadies her head with his right arm and repeats the strokes down the left side of her neck.

He places his hands on Sarah's shoulders and with his right hand he makes three semicircular sweeping movements around the edge of her shoulder blade.

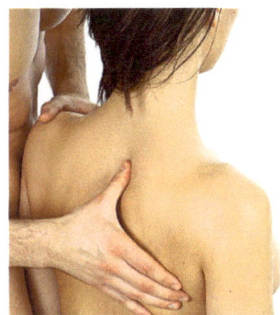

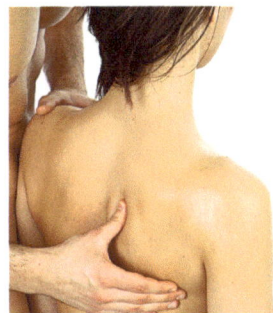

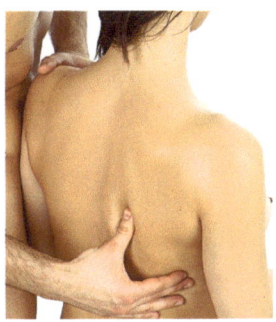

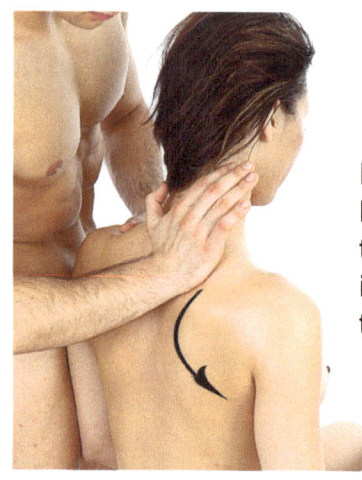

He follows this with horizontal brisk rubbing movements along the edge of the shoulder blade, in a 'C' shape. Repeat this three times.

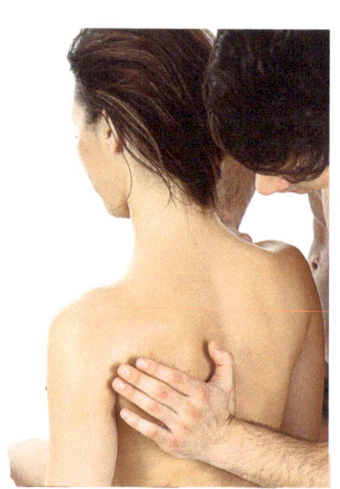

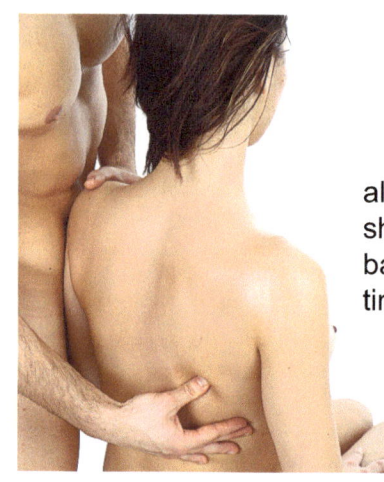

This is followed by a series of circular finger movements along the shoulder blade's edge, which completes the stimulating shoulder blade treatment, helping to break down knots in the back, caused by Sarah's stressful lifestyle. Again, repeat this three times.

James repeats this on the left shoulder and then places both hands on her shoulders again. He kneads and squeezes the shoulder muscles, working from the neck outwards, and back again. He spends some time on this as Sarah has been getting pains in her shoulders lately. He pushes the muscles forwards and backwards, stretching them and working out the knots.

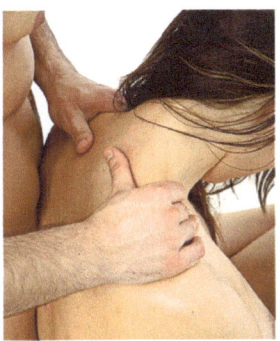 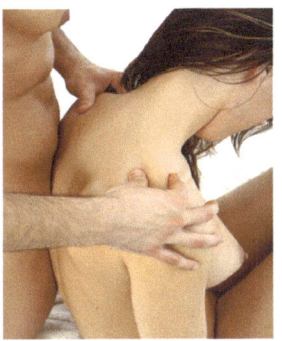 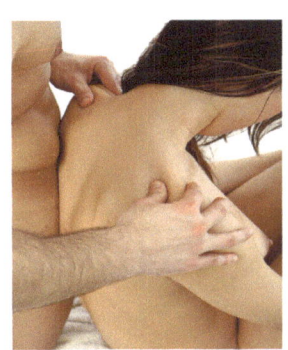

James squeezes the muscle fibres running along Sarah's shoulders, from her neck to her shoulder joint.

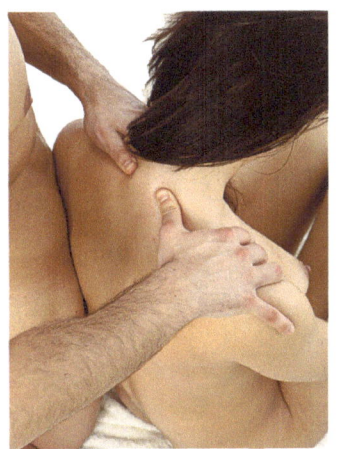

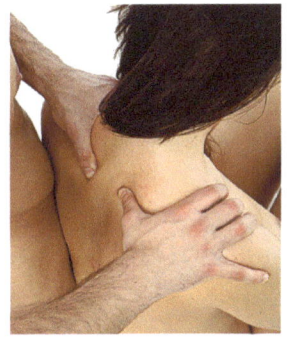

Next, placing his thumbs either side of the spine, at the top of Sarah's shoulders, he pushes firmly either side of the vertebrae, working his way to halfway down her back, at 3cm intervals. This stretches the major trapezius muscle where it attaches diagonally to both sides of the spine.

To finish off the back, James places his hands together in a 'prayer' like position over Sarah's spine and sweeps his hands outwards across her back to her shoulders. This helps to loosen knotty fibres. He repeats this a few more times before giving her loving embrace.

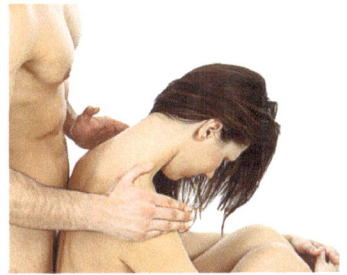 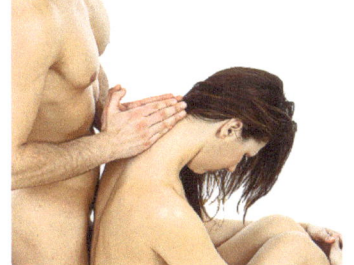 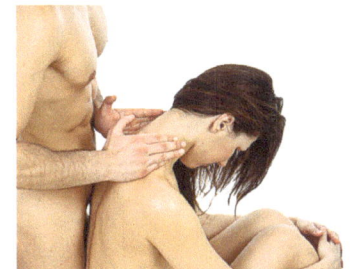

WALKING BAREFOOT TONES THE
MUSCULOSKELETAL STRUCTURE
OF THE FEET

10. MINI MASSAGES - FOOT MASSAGE

If a full body massage is not convenient you could just concentrate on one part of your partner's body. The face, hands and feet are the most sensitive parts of the body, so why not treat your partner to a mini massage?

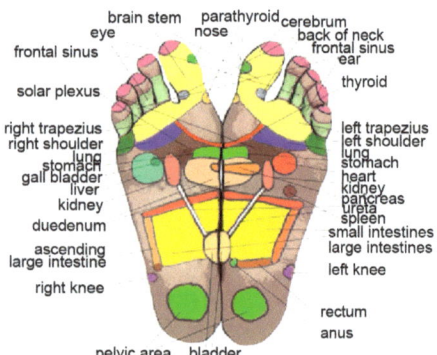

Having your feet massaged can be a blissful experience. Even if your feet are ticklish, it need not put you off. You will soon get used to the firm pressure of your partner's touch. The trick is to have warm firm hands and keep the movements flowing. Don't use cold oils or lotions, and keep your hands on the feet at all times. Try putting your oil mixture in a small bowl and warming it in a pan of hot water for a few minutes.

This diagram shows some of the reflexology points on the soles of the feet. They are thought to be linked to the organs in the body and reflexologists use them to diagnose imbalances in the body's complex system. Pressure is applied to specific areas to encourage healing and balance. You may find some parts of your feet feel tender, hard or gravely. Why not try giving your partner's feet some extra attention and see if they feel the difference.

As with any therapeutic treatment, make sure you have some undisturbed time to yourselves. Put on some soft romantic music, turn down the lights and wash your feet in warm water. Even this can be part of the treatment.

Bring a washing up bowl of warm water and a couple of towels into the room. Put a large towel on the floor and place your bowl of water just in front of your favourite comfy seat. You can put a couple of drops of essential oil in the water to help you relax. Then immerse both feet in the water and let them soak for a little while. Maybe your partner will stroke your feet and rub away dried skin from your heals. Maybe you would like to light a few scented candles and talk over some romantic memories together?

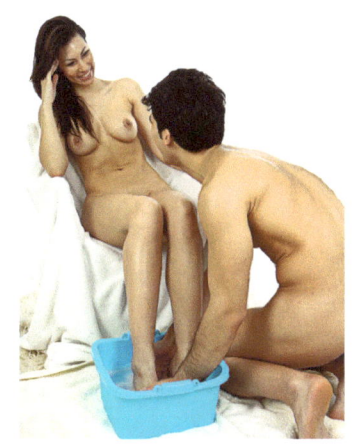

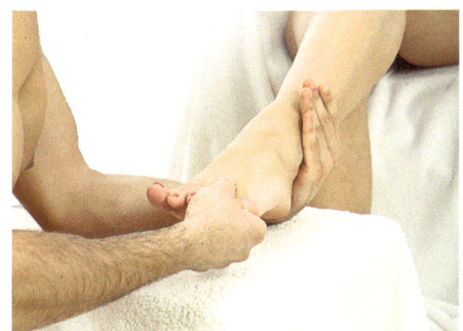

Dry your partner's feet and place a low footstool (or pile of cushions) for her to rest her feet on. Put a towel on the stool to protect it. Sit on a cushion on the floor facing the footstool close enough for you to massage her feet without overstretching. Alternatively, if you have a large couch you could sit, one at each end and have your partner rest her feet on a protected cushion.

For a nice smooth foot massage you will need talcum power, baby cream or oil. If the feet are dry and cracked, olive oil will help to soften the skin. Soaking the feet and regularly rubbing them with a pumice stone will help to soften them. Dry cracked feet can be quite abrasive to your partner's hands, so it is worth keeping them in good condition. Make sure your toenails are not rough and jagged too, as this can scratch his hands.

When you are ready, with warm well-oiled hands, smooth the lubricant over your partner's foot and invigorate them with rubbing strokes either side of the foot. Grasp her foot and slide your hands along to the toes, giving them a gentle stretch

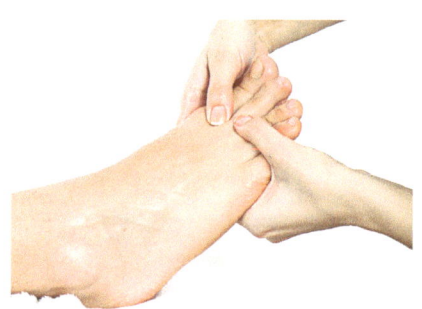

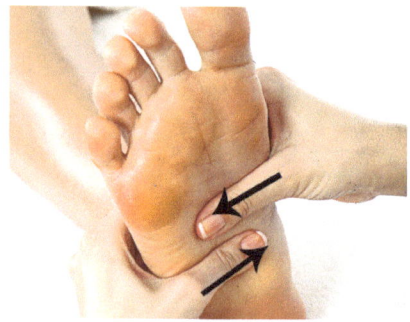

Hold the foot with the sole facing you and fingers over the arch. Move your thumbs with a firm pressure under the foot, moving from the toes to the heels, and back again.

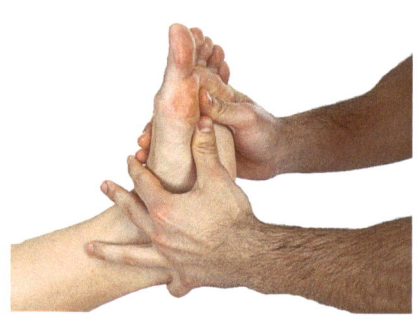

A tender touch is needed for the next movement. With well-oiled fingers grasp each toe in turn and rotate it.

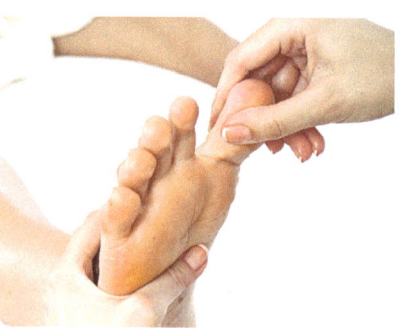

Give each toe a little tug, stretching the muscles and joints.

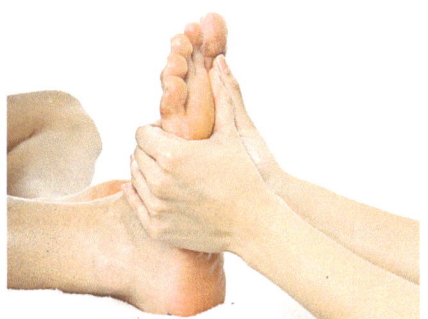

Massage the ball of the foot firmly with your thumbs and work your way under each of the toes.

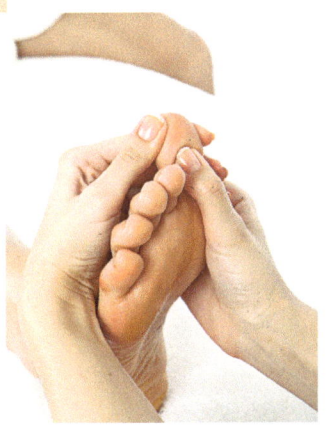

Gently rub the pads of the toes and work your way around the ends of the toes and nails.

Next run your thumbs from the base of each toe, along the tendons and up over the arch to the ankle.

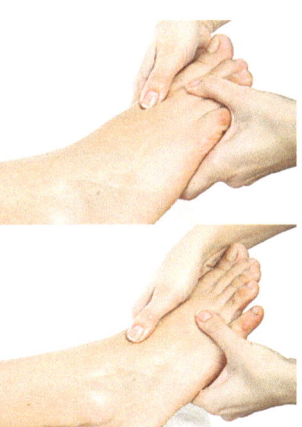

This helps to smooth out the muscle fibres and brings nutrients to them. Repeat this several times

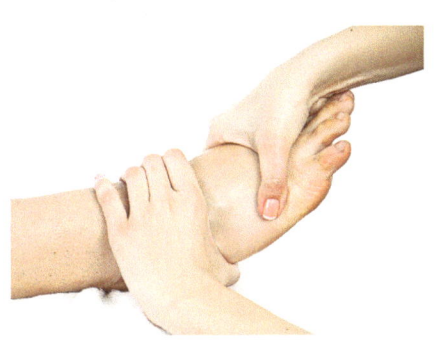

then twist the foot carefully in a wringing motion to help to keep it supple.

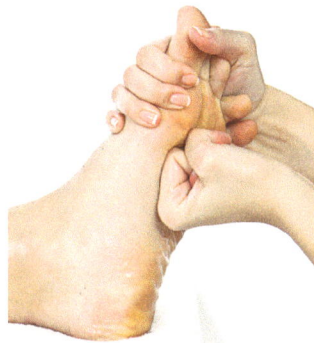

Make a knuckle with your hand and, holding the foot firmly on the top, work your way firmly over the sole.

Rub firmly under the arch of the foot, moving your hand in a circular motion to stimulate all the reflexology points.

Open out your hand and rub under the sole of the foot with the fleshy part of your hand, finishing off around the heel and ankle. Massage firmly around these parts as they get a lot of hard treatment throughout our lives.

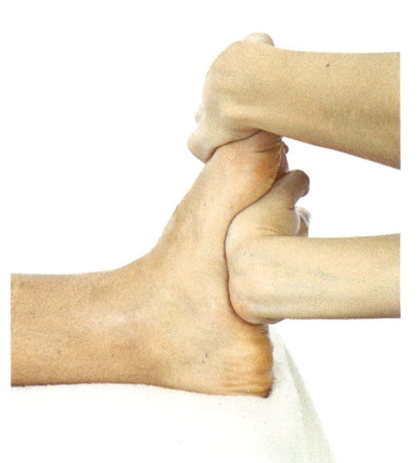

When you have completed one foot, work on the other, then rest together, enjoying the peace and relaxation you have achieved

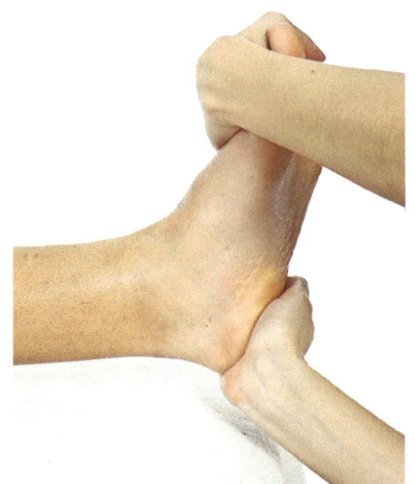

11. MINI MASSAGES - FACE MASSAGE

What better way to instill trust in your partner than to give them a soothing face massage? The face is such a delicate area and is so important to most people. We strive to achieve a healthy complexion, to look young and attractive. Massage can really benefit the complexion as well as bringing about a feeling of relaxation and peace. As in body massage, it stimulates the circulation, elimination of waste products and tones muscles.It is important not to press too hard or overstretch the skin, especially round the eyes. Don't use strong essential oils either, as the skin on the face is thinner and more easily damaged than, say, the hands.

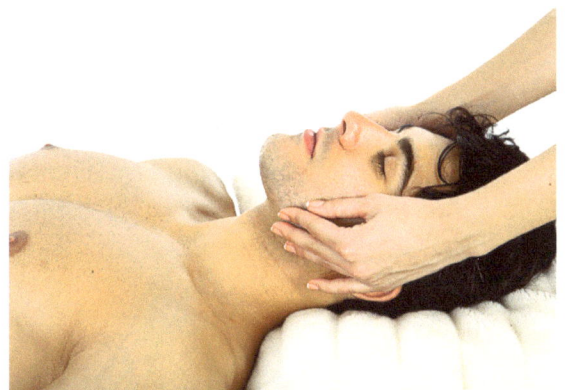

With your partner lying comfortably on the bed, or, with you sitting on the floor with his head cradled in your lap, apply a little cream or lotion to your hands and gentle smooth it over his forehead, cheeks and chin.

Repeat this a few times, then smooth the skin on the forehead in the same direction. Work your fingers in a circular movement over the temples - this movement is very relaxing.

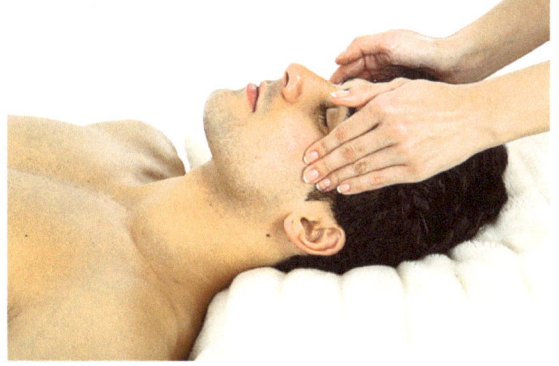

Next, with your fingers well lubricated and using your first and second fingers, press very gently at small intervals, as you work your way across the eyebrows and round the eye sockets. Finish off by tenderly sweeping around the eye sockets, working in the direction of the hairs of the eyebrows.

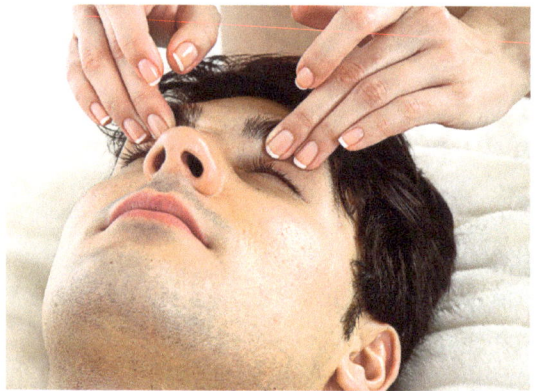
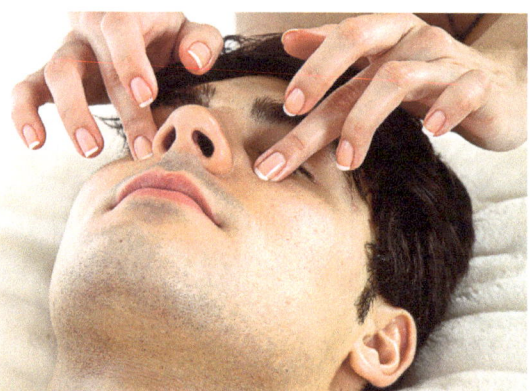

Working over the sinuses and cheek bones can help to increase blood circulation, improve skin and relieve sinus congestion. Again, with well lubricated fingers, place all four fingers of each hand either side of the top of the nose and sweep them across the cheek bones towards the ears. Repeat this several times, pushing the stale blood and lymph towards the lymph nodes around the ear. Give this area a good massage, using firm circular motions.

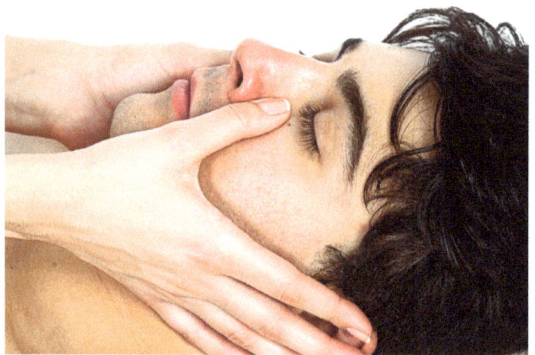
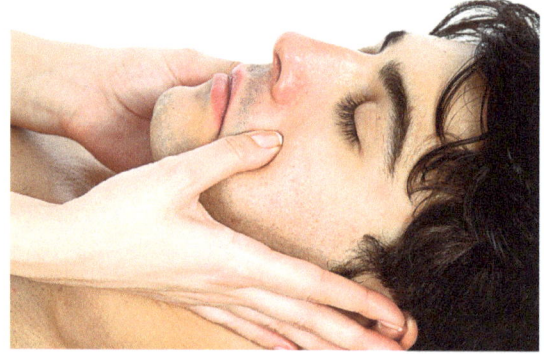

With fingers and thumbs, work your way along the bottom edge of the jaw, starting at the chin, squeezing gently at small intervals until you reach the ears.

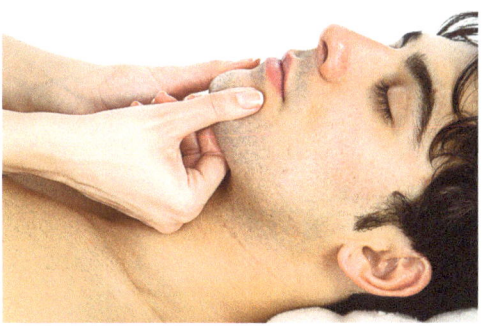

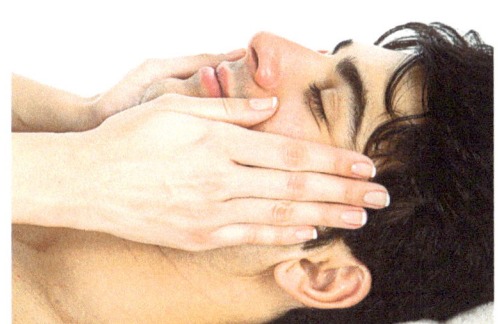

Then flatten both hands and make careful sweeps across the cheeks, from the nose to the ears, working the massage lotion into the skin to give your partner's face a soft glow.

Move gradually round from one side of the neck to the other, always working towards the face and lymph nodes. Repeat this sequence several times …

… and then massage the ear lobes, to finish the face area.

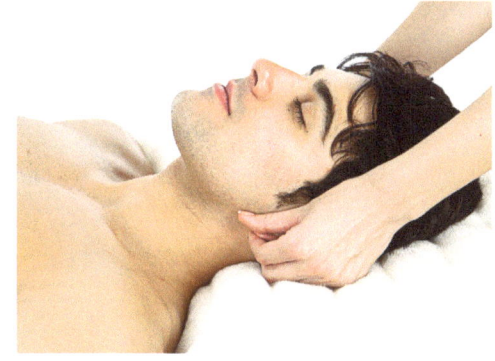

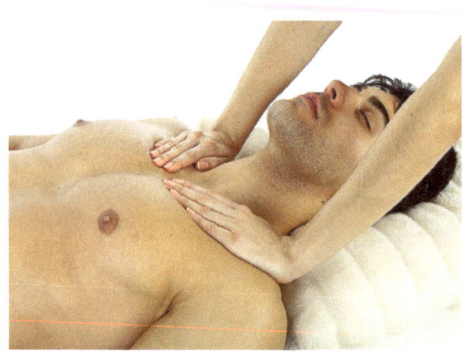

A lovely way to finish the face and neck massage is to sweep the hands across the top of the shoulders, over the collar bones.

Pushing down firmly as you go, stretches the muscles, helping to increase flexibility, reduce stress and drain away waste products.

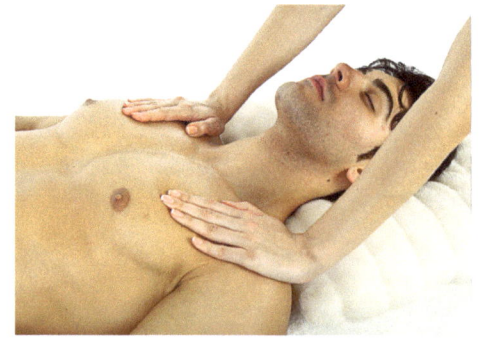

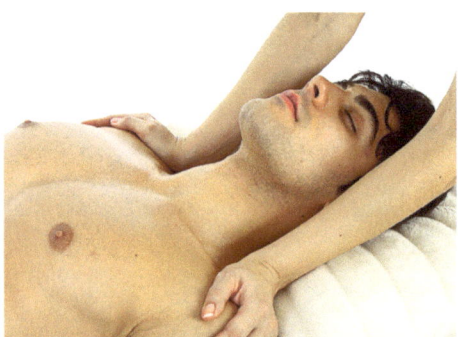

12. ROMANTIC MUTUAL MASSAGE

Once you are familiar with the massage routine it can be really exquisite to share a romantic massage together, as you treat each other simultaneously. You can achieve this lying together on the bed or a cushioned floor. You will need a washable blanket or some large bath towels and you can use oils, lotions, creams or talcum powder.

James and Sarah have decided to have a mutual massage so they can share some loving time together. They have made sure the room was warm, cosy, dimly lit and sweet smelling. Sarah put some scented oils in a burner and lit some of their favourite incense. Lying side by side on the bed they choose their favourite massage lotion containing lavender and ylang ylang. They squeeze some into their hands and rub them together to warm them, ready for their routine.

Step one - one arm

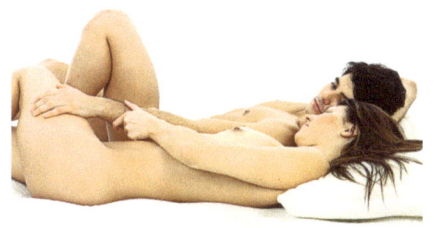

James, with Sarah lying on his left, rests his left arm across Sarah's chest as she lubricates his arm, from his hand up to his shoulder ...

and stroking his arm rhythmically, pulling her hands, one after the other, up towards the top of his arm, working the lotion into his skin and gliding along the fibres of the muscles.

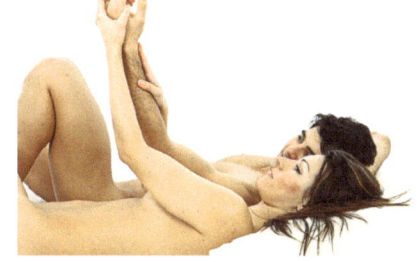

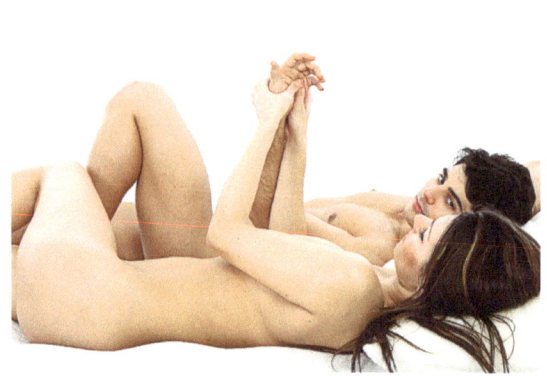

Holding his hand in hers, Sarah firmly massages his fingers, back of his hand and palm. Now it is James' turn to massage Sarah's left arm, as she rests it across his chest.

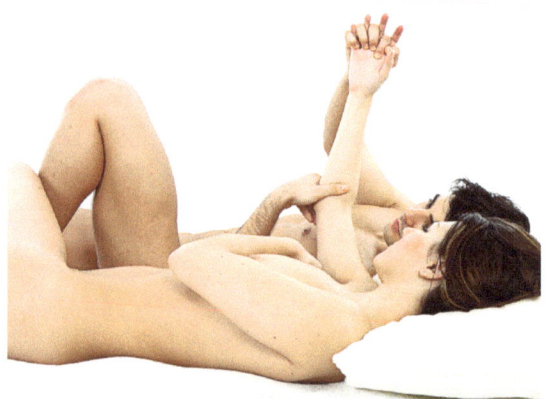

Taking her hand he proceeds to work his way up her arm, being careful to check the pressure of his strokes. He is aware that her arms are not as muscular as his and her skin is more delicate.

Step two – chest and abdomen

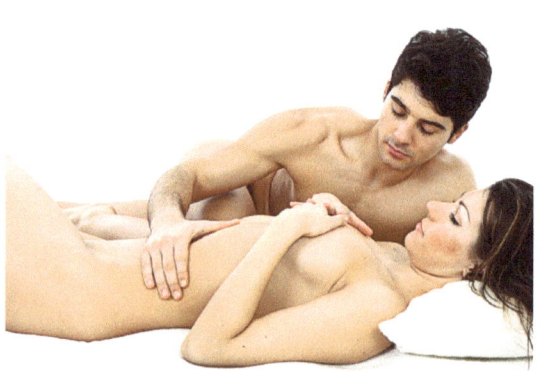

James applies some lotion to Sarah's upper body as he reaches over to massage her abdomen and chest.

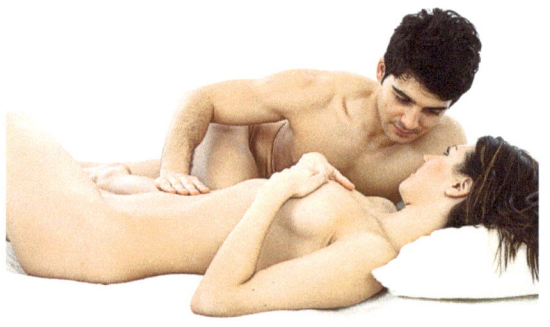

Using his free hand he uses a variety of strokes, remembering to stroke towards the lymph nodes under her arm. He massages her tummy in a clockwise direction towards her groin.

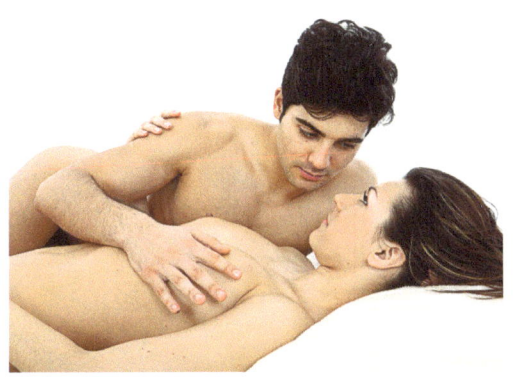

The couple really enjoy this part of the massage and when Sarah has finished James reciprocates. He uses gentle circular movements around her breasts, working towards the armpits.

Sarah is prone to pre-menstrual tension and her breasts are often tender just before a period. Her tummy, too, tends to swell a bit and she finds this massage very helpful.

Step three – both legs

The next part of the routine is on the legs and the couple enjoy treating each other simultaneously. This requires a bit of maneuvering as Sarah swivels round on the bed so she is now at the opposite end. James and Sarah now have each other's feet ready to massage. James and Sarah rest their right legs on each other's body as they oil their hands and works on each other's feet.

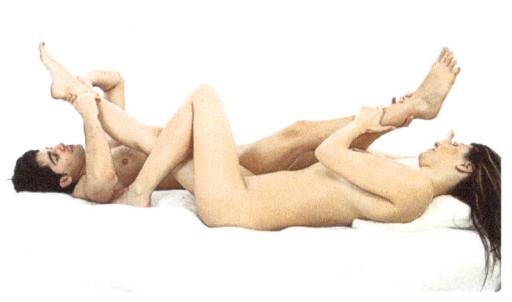

Holding his foot in both hands, Sarah uses firm pressure with her thumbs to work over James' sole. He has recently had a stomach upset and he winces slightly as she works on the pressure point relating to that organ, just below the ball joint of the big toe

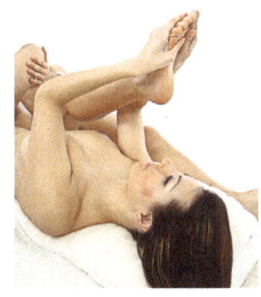

They have both read about reflexology and know that when the soles of the feet are put together you can draw an imaginary 'map' of the body. They have found this to be an effective guide and often use these points to maintain good health. (See chapter 10)

Next they smooth lotion on each other's ankles and calves and work their way up their legs, as far as they can comfortably reach. Sarah maneuvers again to the other side of James' body and they proceed to massage the other leg.

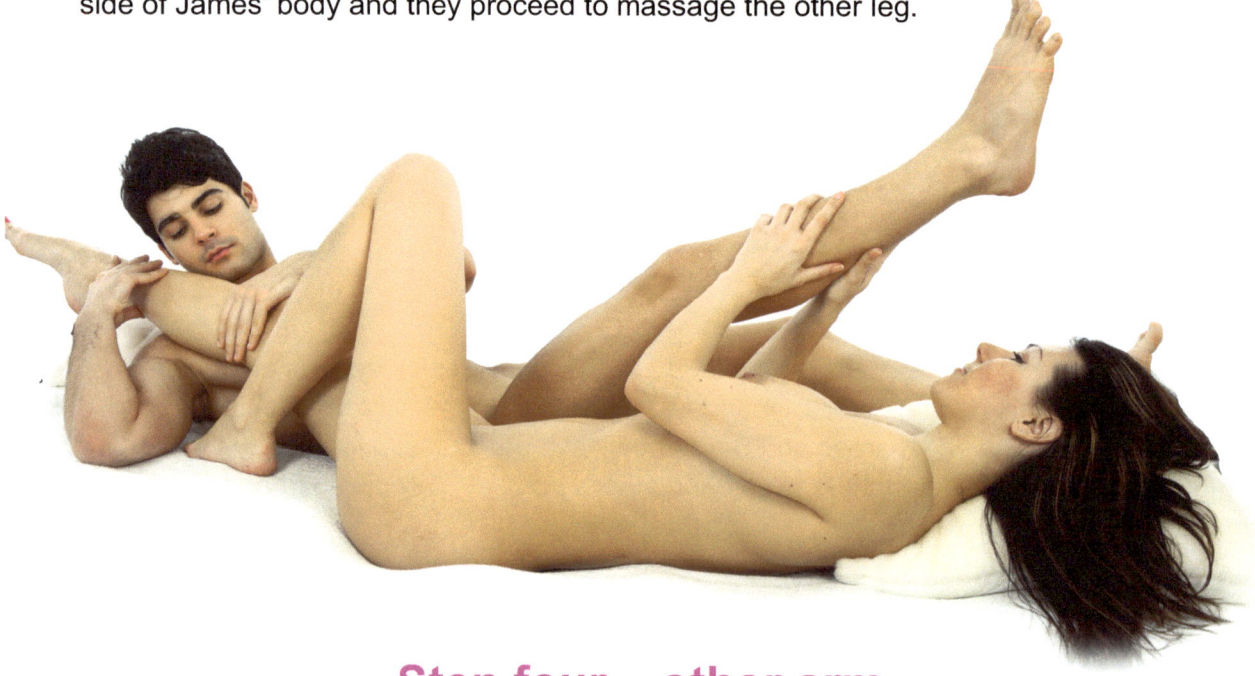

Step four – other arm

Sarah, now on James' right side, turns so that her head is next to his again. She rests her left arm on his chest, as he repeats the arm massage, which was at the beginning of the routine. James rests his arm on Sarah's chest and she massages his left arm.

Step five – back massage

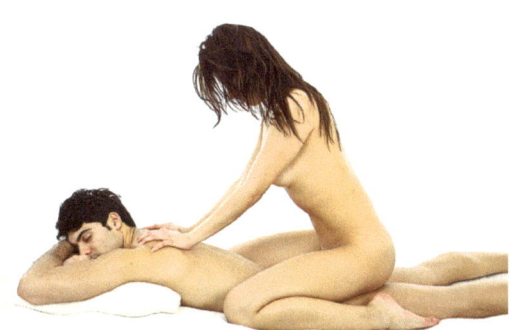

James turns over onto his front and Sarah straddles James for the last part of the routine. She pours some lotion into her hands, rubs them together, and massages her partner's back. She uses long firm strokes across his shoulders and down his back and spends some time squeezing and rubbing his shoulder and neck muscles.

Lastly she turns round, still straddling James, so that she is facing his feet. She firmly massages James' buttocks and upper thighs, following the line of the large bundles of muscles.

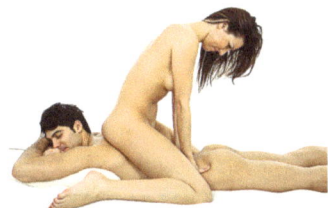

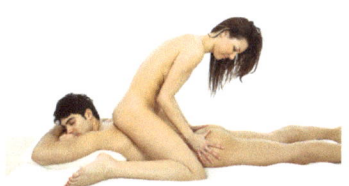

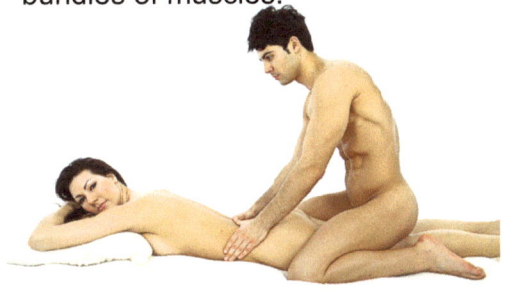

The soft bed helps to spread the weight and using this position they can give each other the maximum benefit of the massage.

When they have finished they feel relaxed and warm. They have a refreshing drink and then cuddle up together to enjoy the peace and harmony they have created.

I TRUST YOU TO BE KIND AND GENTLE.

I SHARE EVERY ASPECT OF MY BODY

WITH YOU. I AM LIKE A BABY IN

YOUR TENDER CARE

13. MASSAGE YOUR RELATIONSHIP

An elderly devoted couple, when asked recently the reason for the success of their sixty years of marriage, replied 'share everything, the good and the bad. Talk, talk, talk. Never go to bed on an argument, even if it means staying up all night. Cry together, laugh together, share your intimate thoughts and feelings and above all, work hard to make your marriage work. We all change as we grow older, you must change together or you will drift apart'.

Many relationships are different now, far less firmly cemented together. Same sex relationships are accepted and acceptable, there is more sexual freedom, and it is easier for people to leave a difficult marriage. Perhaps there is not such a strong incentive for people to stay together, as wives are no longer totally dependent on their husbands for an income and place to live, and there is more temptation in the workplace. However, the fluidity of relationships can be harmful for the children, as they lose their stability in life and grow up confused and disturbed.

Very few relationships are 'made in heaven', everyone has different thoughts and opinions, and very few people agree all the time. We come back to the importance of physical touch, taking us emotionally back to our roots as tiny babies. Allowing ourselves be intimately touched is to be vulnerable, to be vulnerable is to trust, and trust is a vital part of a good relationship.

By giving a gentle massage you are saving to your partner 'trust me not to hurt you or criticise your body'. By accepting massage you are saying 'I trust you to be kind and gentle, I share every aspect of my body with you, I am like a baby in your tender care'.

The intimate side of a relationship can often be affected by many problems. Stress, anger, jealousy, tiredness and many other emotions, can come between, what should be, a natural expression of love between two people. What better way to ease these problems than to share a wonderful massage? Make yourself vulnerable to your partner and learn to trust each other again.

> RELAX AND SENSE THE LIFE WITHIN YOU. BE AWARE THAT EVERYTHING IS BEING TAKEN CARE OF - YOU ARE UNIQUE AND SPECIAL.

14. HEIGHTENING YOUR SENSES

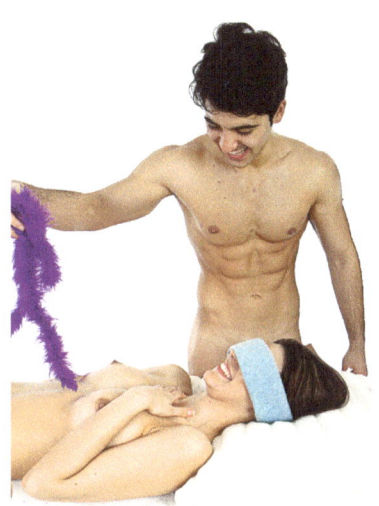

I have emphasised the importance of atmosphere when you share your massage time together. This is because the more external influences there are, the less you will appreciate the tactile experiences. Out of your five senses, touch is the most important for your emotional wellbeing. Keep the volume of any background music low, just above hearing level. Dim the lights and use gentle, natural fragrances. By decreasing external stimuli you will savour your partner's loving touch, your nervous system will remain calm and you will feel delicious.

To heighten your senses, why not try stroking a feather over your partner's body? Using a blindfold will further add to the sensations. Anything soft, such as cotton wool or a silk scarf will be effective.

You could also try feeding your partner. Keep the blindfold on and pop some fruit or a small piece of chocolate in her mouth. Or try a kiss - anywhere on the body - keep her guessing. (Remember to use natural edible oils for your massage!)

ENJOY!

15. ESSENTIAL OILS TO ENHANCE YOUR RELATIONSHIP

Stress
Basil, camomile, jasmine, lavender, lemon, marjoram, neroli, orange, peppermint, petitigrain, rose, sage, tangerine, vetivert, ylang ylang.

Mood swings
Basil, bay, cajuput, camomile, incense, lavender, lemon, marjoram, neroli, orange, peppermint, petitgrain, tangerine, vetivert, ylang ylang

Anger
Jasmine, lavender, marjoram, neroli, petitgrain, Roman camomile, tangerine, vetivert.

Frigidity
Incense, jasmine, juniper, lavender, neroli, orange, ylang ylang

Jealousy
Jasmine, juniper, lavender, marjoram, peppermint, petitgrain, Roman camomile, vetivert, ylang ylang

Tiredness
Bay, bergamot, incense, jasmine, juniper, orange, petitgrain, rose, rosemary

Depression
Bay, bergamot, black pepper, cajuput, jasmine, marjoram, orange, petitgrain, rose, tangerine, thyme

Poor immunity
Bay basis, cajuput, eucalyptus, geranium, lavender, lemon, myrrh, orange, pine, thyme

Worry
Bergamot, jasmine, marjoram, neroli, incense, orange, peppermint, petitgrain, Roman camomile, rose, tangerine, thyme, vetivert, ylang ylang

Stiff and achy
Black pepper, cajuput, cypress, eucalyptus, juniper, marjoram, lavender, lemon, orange, pine, rosemary, sage, thyme

Poor appetite
Bergamot, black pepper, juniper, myrrh, neroli, peppermint, Roman camomile, rosemary, sage, thyme

Blood pressure
Lavender, lemon, petitgrain, rose, ylang ylang

Sleep problems
Lavender, marjoram, petitgrain, rose, thyme, vetivert, ylang ylang

ABOUT THE AUTHOR

I have worked as a complementary therapist for many years and have a practice in Buckinghamshire, UK. I became interested in health issues over thirty years ago, when my own health problems would not respond to conventional medicine.

I was introduced to a spiritual healer and was amazed to find that the problem improved dramatically. I eventually became a healer myself and went on to investigate the many different complementary therapies on offer.

I am passionate about healthy living and leading a natural life and have written many articles and booklets on diet and health. You may also wish to read my newly published book

Why Sugar Makes You Hungry And Dieting Makes You Fat.

I also studied hypnosis and its effect on health. I teach meditation, relaxation and healing and also enjoy writing music. I found that there was very little appropriate therapeutic music. It needs to be musical but not memorable, slow, harmonious and without a beat. Drum beats can affect the heart rate. Being a musician, I decided to write and record my own relaxation music, specifically to calm the mind. With my husband's help we have now published it as a CD, with a short calming narrative at the beginning. My 'Inner Harmony' CD has been very successful and I still use it on a regular basis.

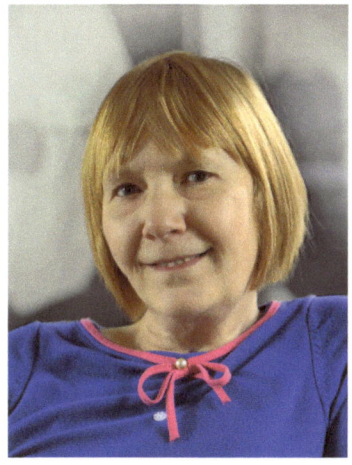

Inner Harmony CD – meditation and relaxation to calm the mind and body